The Real Deal Guide to Pregnancy

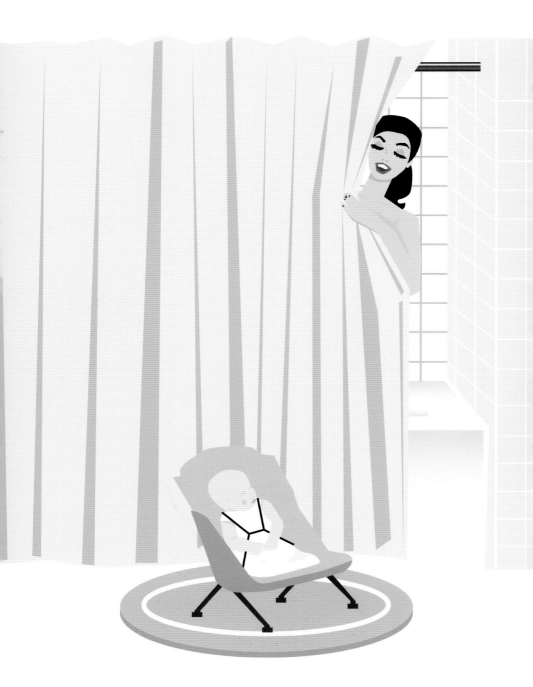

The Real Deal Guide to Pregnancy

Fresh and Practical Advice
for Navigating the Next
Nine Months

Erika Lenkert

London, New York,
Mellbourne, Munich and Delhi

Senior Editor Anja Schmidt
Editorial Assistant Nichole Morford
Managing Art Editor Michelle Baxter
Art Director Dirk Kaufman
DTP Coordinator Kathy Farias
Production Manager Ivor Parker
Executive Managing Editor Sharon Lucas

Illustrations by Diana Catherines /Design Design

First American Edition, 2008

Published in the United States by
DK Publishing
375 Hudson Street, New York, New York 10014
08 09 10 11 12 10 9 8 7 6 5 4 3 2 1
PD205—March 2008
Copyright © 2008 Dorling Kindersley Limited
Text copyright © 2008 Erika Lenkert
All rights reserved

A catalog record for this book is available from the
Library of Congress.
ISBN 978-0-7566-3386-8

DK books are available at special discounts when
purchased in bulk for sales promotions, premiums,
fund-raising, or educational use. For details, contact:
DK Publishing Special Markets, 375 Hudson Street,
New York, New York 10014 or SpecialSales@dk.com.

Printed and bound in China by Hung Hing

Discover more at
www.dk.com

Neither the publisher nor the author is engaged in rendering professional advice or
services to the individual reader. The ideas, procedures, and suggestions contained
in this book are not intended as a substitute for consulting with your physician.
All matters regarding your health require medical supervision. Neither the author
nor the publisher shall be liable or responsible for any loss or damage allegedly
arising from any information or suggestion in this book.

This book is dedicated to Viva, my miraculous, fearless,
funny, and eternally joyful girl. Life with her makes all the
sacrifices of motherhood my greatest privilege and honor.

CONTENTS

One day I was expertly powering through my busy-girl life. The next day, during a morning bathroom run, a little plastic stick emblazoned with a "+" turned me into a clueless wonder who didn't know how to maneuver through her own every-day world. Like most newly pregnant women, I dashed to the nearest bookstore for guidance and bought all the standard pregnancy books. But as I read through them I discovered that no one resource covered what I—and apparently all of my mommy friends—wanted when we got pregnant: a book that condensed all of the essential topics into a fun and factual, easy-to-read, quick-resource guide couched in everyday practicality and packed with must-have information, empathy, and ways to compare our experience with that of others.

So I decided to write the book we wanted to read.

You're holding the results in your hands. A frank, upbeat, CliffsNotes-like handbook, this guide will not force you to read endlessly to find the one morsel of information you need, scare the bejeezus out of you with every possible pregnancy scenario, or answer every single medical question you have (although you will find a plethora of first-hand pregnancy experiences and tons of concrete, medically approved advice). It was written to quickly arm you with everyday essentials on how to sashay, and later waddle, your way through maternity's everyday realities and maladies—and know that you're not alone when you cry at corny commercials, hurl at the smell of coffee, or look down one day and discover that your ankles are now as wide and doughy as your knees.

Within the following pages you'll find important facts on food, exercise, and medical minutiae, and advice on how to heighten your sleep, self-esteem, and pamper potential. You'll also discover stupidly easy, but extremely important, tips on how to remedy, or at least manage, unpleasant pregnancy symptoms, and deepen and enrich your relationship with your partner—even if that seems about as likely right now as fitting into your tightest pair of jeans. Other bonuses include fashion advice, sex stats, reviews of books, shops, and online maternity resources, details on how to prepare for the big day and beyond, and enough of my own gestational adventures to make you more in the know than my OB-GYN.

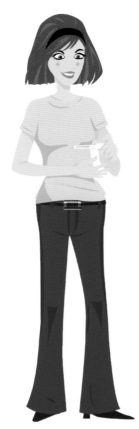

But this book isn't filled merely with hard facts, sound advice, and my own pregnancy particulars. Since every pregnancy is different, I wanted to offer the widest variety of pregnancy experiences, perspectives, and tips, so I enlisted 111 pregnant women and moms from around the country and abroad, aged from 18 to 45 at the time that they were pregnant, to fill out a laborious, confidential 68-question survey. Referred to throughout the book as the Mommy Menagerie, these miraculous women (who between them now have at least 183 children) provided the information and insight they wish someone had shared with them, as well as enough facts and figures to fill this book with spectacular statistics, polls, and stories. You will find their quotes everywhere, without attribution to protect their confidentiality and trust. Check out the acknowledgments on page 255 for a list of these fabulously insightful females. Thanks to them I believe that this guide truly is an invaluable resource and the absolute real deal.

One word about semantics: Just as every pregnancy is different, so are every woman's medical preferences and circumstances. To keep things simple I use the term "practitioner" and "doctor" in this book to describe maternity professionals, whether it's an OB-GYN or a midwife (although midwives aren't technically doctors). Similarly, "partner" can translate to whomever is in your life that is going through this experience with you, bearing the brunt of any hormonal tirades, and fetching chicken tacos upon demand.

Now, go on with your fabulous pregnant self, and read ahead for your first heaping helping of insight from the Mommy Menagerie, who selflessly served up what they would do differently if they got pregnant again so that others might learn from their trimesters of trial and error.

The Mommy Menagerie On ...Hindsight

When asked, "What would you do differently if there were to be a next time?" mommies had myriad answers, ranging from nothing to everything. Me? I'd try to avoid any edible indulgences for as long as possible since one bite of a cookie opens the carb-and-sugar floodgates. I'd also do lots of yoga, strive harder for a vaginal birth, set up childcare in advance, and prepare and address my birth announcements before the B-day. Check out what other mommies mentioned:

"I am pregnant again so I'm able to act on this now. I think I am allowing myself to not be as nervous. I realize now that no matter how much we worry, there usually isn't anything we can do about how a pregnancy goes, so all worry does is make it worse for both the mother and the baby."

"Now I know I will get fat, so I won't be so afraid of it."

"I would enjoy and appreciate my pregnant body. A pregnant woman is the most beautiful sight. I just couldn't see the beauty in my own body. Next time I will relish it."

"I would eat better. I think I allowed myself to splurge a little too much."

"Eat what I wanted, regardless of medical advice—women have been having babies for a long time and should learn to trust their bodies more!"

"Eat iron-fortified breakfast cereal throughout pregnancy."

"Eat and try to gain more weight (not from junk food but a healthy diet) earlier in the pregnancy."

"Enjoy it more, not work as hard."

"I think I would try to control the outbursts a little more."

"Say NO to extraneous activities and rest more."

"Give up any ideas of being Superwoman and allow others to help me."

"Funny, but all the things I would do differently (get more sleep, read a book about parenting—not just pregnancy— buy stuff sooner) won't be possible the next time around!"

"This is the next time and I'm doing the same thing . . . taking it one day at a time."

"I am pregnant for the second time now, and I am much more relaxed this time around. I know what to do and not to do. I don't spend a lot of time searching for the right things to eat, wear, and worrying about what I can and cannot do."

"I would take pictures of my naked belly and body, which I didn't do at all the first time, and I would keep a daily journal."

"I would take a fantastic vacation in the second trimester, rather than the third."

"Try to pamper myself more...take more naps, relax more."

"Sleep more."

"Get more pregnancy massages! No guilt for the expense—I'd build it into the budget. It's that worth it."

"Avoid going into any maternity clothing stores until I need a pair of jeans. I really want to avoid spending money on maternity clothes and instead save money until after the baby comes and buy something that I will actually get to wear for a long time."

"Buy some cuter clothes."

"I'd be in better shape at the beginning and I'd spend half an hour in the gym every day."

"Swim."

"Use the elliptical trainer more."

"I would not work as much and spend more time remembering every detail of the pregnancy."

"Read less and go more by instinct."

"Not tell anyone the names or sex of the baby until it is born. Difficult to do, but it would have saved a lot of grief."

"I would get together with more pregnant ladies so that we could exchange experiences, like a pregnant woman's support group. There were so many things [going on that] no one could understand what you were going through unless they were pregnant with you. I spent some time on online support groups, but you definitely need human contact for support as well."

"Be more open with my husband about my feelings and what I needed from him."

"Not think that because my husband wasn't interested in my pregnancy that it meant he would not be a good, interested, devoted dad."

"I would never be pregnant during the summer again!"

"I might start earlier than 35!"

"Request an ultrasound earlier—we didn't find out until 12 weeks that we had twins!"

"Get a doula!"

"I hope to not have an epidural this time."

"Have a midwife at my labor instead of a doctor/hospital setting."

"The next time I would love to do a water birth, although I'm now considered high risk, which makes it difficult."

"Have the baby at home."

"Try to enjoy it more rather than feel so tired and sick and resent that part of it. I'm someone who really needs to feel physically good all the time or it makes me feel depressed that I'm not healthy. I don't always see the light at the end of the tunnel—I forget that things are temporary."

"Not freak out as much, especially about things like 'I do not want to poo on the delivery table.' Who cares? Just get the kid out!"

"Enjoy the time because it goes fast."

Personal Pregnancy Timeline

2 weeks: My boobs look like I had instant breast enlargement surgery; they hurt so much that blowing on them is almost painful. I don't know I'm pregnant, but have a hunch.

3 weeks: An insatiable craving for bacon hits. It lasts for one week and includes four packs of nitrite-free slabs. After that, I just want to eat all of everything—for the next two months.

4 weeks: The test confirms my suspicion! I panic, wondering if I'm doing everything wrong, buy books, comb the web, and finally relax and remember that women have been doing this for centuries without a manual. I also continue my half hour runs and light weights.

6 weeks: I begin waking up every night at 3am and staring at the wall for a solid hour before falling back to sleep. This lasts three weeks.

8 weeks: I become stupidly exhausted, sometimes waking up feeling more tired than when I went to sleep. I know on those days I'm worthless and now empathize with children who scream and cry with overtiredness. I have become one of them. Thankfully there's the occasional respite. This lasts four weeks. Gotta pee in the middle of the night all the time; this lasts a month then disappears for my entire second trimester.

9 weeks: My yoo-hoo itches like a son of a gun! I bathe excessively, wear cotton undies, and use a topical cream until I freak and find out the manufacturer warns against using it without consulting my doctor. My doctor says everything in the world warns against use during pregnancy (we're a sue-happy nation, after all), and says it's okay. (That said, check with your doctor before using any yoo-hoo helpers!) It occasionally itches throughout the rest of my pregnancy.

10 weeks: I've gained 10 pounds and those annoying books say I'm supposed to gain 5 at the most. I stop reading and keep eating.

12 weeks: What "they" say is true! My exhaustion disappears and now I'm on top of the world—and hurrying to do everything in fear that it's very temporary. Turns out it's not! I am Superwoman for the rest of my pregnancy. Woo-hoo!

13 weeks: It doesn't feel right to me to run anymore. I take up brisk walking to disco hits and hard rock on the Treadmill.

14 weeks: I can only fit into one pair of my old pants—a trusty pair of jeans. I wear them every day that I'm not in sweats. Luckily, I'm working from home, but that's about to change.

16 weeks: I finally "pop" so I now look more like a pregnant woman than a hussy with a boob job and a beer belly. I get on the scale at the doctor and see that I'm now 15 pounds heavier. The nurse, who nudges the scale-reading thingy further to the right than I've ever seen it go in my life, cheerily says, "Yippee! You've gained weight!" I'm absolutely positive she's been coached to do that—and I'm grateful. Also got two batches of weird veins on my right inner thigh just above my knee. Looks like a bruise, but is definitely more permanent. My doctor says they'll shrink to the point that they're barely noticeable after the birth (she turns out to be right).

17 weeks: I get an amniocentesis and find out we're having a healthy girl. The next day she announces her arrival with her first no-ticeable movement. It's not a "flutter" like "they" say it will be, but rather a full field-goal kick. I put my hand on my stomach and she does it again. It creeps me out—at least the first time. Definitely like feeling an alien inside you and seeing it trying to get out from the outside. After that I'm used to it, anticipating it, and waiting for her to let me know she's alive and kicking.

18 weeks: Protesting about buying expensive "fat me" clothes, I go to Old Navy and buy three T-shirts and two pairs of pants. I return the pants the next day because the low-waist elastic doesn't work and every time I bend over I get plumber's crack. I'm still in sweats and the trusty old pair of jeans.

19 weeks: Sciatica, or blood-curdling, knee-buckling, hysteria-inducing bouts of lower back pain, which also shoots pain down my legs, begins. I whimper, wince, and complain a lot. I also get stuck on the couch—"I've fallen and I can't get up—seriously!"—and have to call a friend to come rescue me. (My husband Colie is at work an hour away.)

20 weeks: I see a "non-force" chiropractor. He's my new hero. I also notice that when I sit down without a good bra on, my boobs now rest on my belly. It's rather disconcerting. I buy a new bra—a 34D instead of my pre-pregnancy 34B or small C. While shopping for it I realize that for the first time in my life I have big nipples. They seem foreign, like they belong to someone else. I get on the scale at the gym and see that I've gained 20 pounds. I wish the nurse were there to cheer me on.

22 weeks: I give in and go to Pea in the Pod. I spend a small fortune on two bras, three pairs of hip, trendy pants, one black cocktail dress, and three shirts. Only when I get home do I find they forgot to put one pair of pants in the bag. Good thing as the first time I put on my new cute pair of Joie khaki jeans the band rips. The other pair is woefully uncomfortable. Duh! Now I have to make another trip downtown with my round self to return them—for credit only, which I argue against until they give in. The baby moves around all the time now. My husband can't feel it and is frustrated and beginning to lose interest and seems very disappointed. I reassure him that Viva, our girl, needs to get familiar with his touch. After a few ill-fated attempts she wiggles for him—regularly.

24 weeks: I take a business-and-pleasure trip to New York City. After a day of tromping up and down Manhattan's streets I look down and see my ankles have bloated to match the width of my calves. It's not a nice look. I kick up my feet and the swelling goes down.

28 weeks: My back goes out again. I am in so much pain at the doctor's office it takes me 10 minutes to get off of the table—and I'm bawling the whole time. My doctor prescribes Vicodin, which I take twice, when the pain is too much to bear. The unsuccessful chiropractor is no longer my hero. My new savior becomes a registered nurse/body worker who charges a fortune for weekly hour-and-a-half massages, but tweaks my balloon body into comfortable submission. I see her regularly until my due date.

31 weeks: I have a slow subterranean drip and fear my water is leaking. I head to the doctor's office and she tells me I have the worst yeast infection she has ever seen. Despite my competitive nature I do not feel particularly proud. She writes me a prescription for over-the-counter Monistat and sends me on my way. I've gained a lofty 32 pounds now and am excited for the time when the baby is so big I'll always feel full; that time never comes.

35 weeks: I'm waddling around at work, have abandoned all shoes but my running shoes and flip flops, and talk with a windedness that makes me sound like I just ran a marathon. However, the only dashes I make are to the company cookie jar. The baby's room is coming together and I find new reasons to love Target. They have everything.

38 weeks: I can't bear to try to look decent any longer. I'm just too darned big. I begin working at home where no one will know that I am living in low-hanging shorts and T-shirts and regularly require being hoisted out of bed. Still, my weight gain has hit a plateau. I am a hefty 162 pounds and only add one more by the time I hit the maternity ward.

40+ weeks: I've been told that the minute you clear your plate of everything you wanted to get done before you have the baby is when you go into labor. Four days past my due date I press "send" on an e-mail that includes the last piece of business I had to accomplish. Within minutes the fun and games begin (more on this later).

The minute I learned I was pregnant I did what most pregnant gals do: invested in books. My mommy girlfriends warned me to buy only one since most of the guides tend to, among other things, pontificate on the myriad potential pregnancy problems and underscore completely unrealistic dietary guidelines (0 to 5 pound weight gain the first trimester? Once a week treats? Try closer to 12 pounds. And who in their right mind thinks that a healthy and now ever-hungry pregnant woman is going to have the strength or desire to eliminate dessert all but once a week?)

While some of these books have real and useful information, they can make even the healthiest expecting woman insane with worry and weight-scale sagas.

Of course I bought about 10 books anyway, a few of which focused on the down and dirty details and others that highlighted diets and recipes, exercise, and empathy-humor. But I quickly lost interest in all but the breezy pregnancy-humor books. The others weren't fun, happy, "you-go-girl" guides, which are much needed since even the most welcome and expected pregnancies have elements about them that are funky fearful, or downright awful. And besides, the idea of militantly ingesting four servings of vegetables and three of fruit per day was laughable to a well-balanced, prenatal vitamin-popping nibbler like me.

I became overwhelmed and felt that in this case, too much information was too much information. I was glad I had a technical book around for when something weird or new happened and I needed somewhere to turn. But I would encourage you to limit your purchases to one solid encyclopedic baby book (see "Sources," page 238 for suggestions), get additional details online ("Sources" lists some good websites), make lists of questions for your doctor as they arise, and spend the money you saved on something nice for yourself—like a mani-pedi, new cozy PJs, or a facial.

In retrospect, the majority of my reading time would have been better spent on post-pregnancy topics such as breastfeeding—by far the most challenging part of having a baby for me—designing healthy sleep routines for baby, and the realities of the transition to parenthood. These new-mommy navigations made delivery-room contractions and C-section recovery seem like a tea party. Take it from someone who knows: Four months into sleep deprivation and relentless servitude isn't the ideal time to begin researching how to get your depleting milk production back up or cajole your little lovebug into sleeping for more than two hours at a time.

WHAT DO YOU DO NOW?

Whether it is a pleasant surprise or a result of years of planning, when pregnancy hits infinite questions and quandaries immediately follow. For me they started with predictable puzzlements like, "What about the champagne I threw back on our vacation?" "Are my tight pants still safe to wear?" "Are my daily morning runs, hair and beauty products, and mani-pedis dangerous?" "Are hot baths—with bubbles—kosher?" "What shouldn't I eat?" and "Can I safely have sex, and if so, is it okay to use lubricant?"

And then there are the mental and physical changes. If they haven't started already, you're bound to begin feeling some pretty peculiar things and at first not know what to do about them. My second month kicked off with insatiable hunger, soap opera-worthy weepiness, and wide-eyed and inexplicable hour-long wakeups each night at 3am. If you haven't experienced these treats, don't get anxious just yet—symptoms are different for everyone and besides, they are bound to change just as soon as you get used to them. (Incidentally, the same can be said for any sleep schedules, behaviors, and rhythms of your baby once he or she is born.)

It only gets more exciting—and weird—from here, so brace yourself, kick up your feet, pour yourself a tall glass

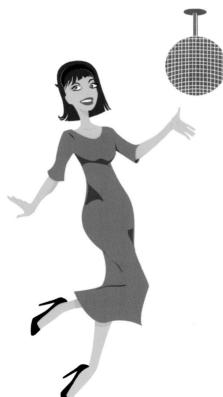

of water—especially since now you should be drinking it like it's your job—and read on for fast facts on what you need to know right now. Once you get through this chapter you'll have answers to many of your immediate questions. Then you can flip through subsequent sections—which give tons of comforting tips as well as greater detail on many of the cheat sheets listed in this chapter—when you're in the mood to know more.

Celebrate!

You now know why perhaps your pants haven't quite fit like they normally do, you've gotten teary-eyed and defensive over things that you'd usually shrug off, or you've been dumping everything in reach into your mouth and you still feel hungry, or are having other unusual reactions. (Most of my mommy friends never experienced morning sickness, myself included, and thought there was something wrong since pregnancy books often talk about it like it's a right of passage.) In any case, relax. You're bound to have your own pregnancy experiences, and even when they are about as fun as slamming your hand in a door, there's comfort in knowing your body is going Exorcist on you for a good reason. Besides, even the creepiest stuff—and trust me there will be some— is nothing short of fascinating and best of all, temporary! So try not to stress over the newness and initial fears of anything and everything going wrong. Put on your favorite disco tune, and do at least one party dance around the living room. After all, you're going to have a baby!

Don't panic about past behavior.

Before you begin freaking out about every little thing you did before you knew you were toting a soon-to-be tot, relax. Every book and doctor will tell you not to worry about yesterday's cocktails and sushi extravaganza or the cigarette you smoked last night. Besides, it's too late to do anything about it anyway. But if you want a little reassurance, just reflect on a few generations ago when cigarettes and martinis were a common part of a pregnancy diet. Or remember that lots of people get in a family way as a result of a freewheeling night on the town or a New Year's romp. In my case it was a little of all of the above: a romantic vacation complete with raw sushi, free-flowing champagne, and sleep-inducing melatonin pills for the 14-hour plane ride home, followed by a long weekend of Thanksgiving toasts, unabashed gluttony, and hard workouts at the gym. And nine months later I had a healthy baby girl. That said, now that you know you're pregnant, it is a good idea to start acting like it.

When to Behave

The first trimester is when your baby's organs are developing, so it's the most important time to lay off the no-nos as best you can.

If you haven't already,

begin taking prenatal vitamins. Not only do they provide you with very important nutritional necessities for your growing baby, they also might make you feel a little less guilty if all you can manage to keep down is that tub of ice cream you just inhaled.

Unfortunately, deciding to take them is easier than picking which brand to pop for the next nine-plus months. Step up to the vitamin section at the drugstore, or better yet health food store, and you'll be faced with enough choices to make your already sensitive stomach turn. Making the decision more frustrating is that the FDA does not regulate what goes into prenatal vitamins so all options are not created equal. But don't sweat it—it's not as though companies out there are trying to create bad vitamins. You just want to get the most pill for your pop—especially since their gargantuan size makes swallowing them a really special experience.

Call your regular doctor and ask for over-the-counter or prescription suggestions for pills that pack the healthiest wallop. Or, if you go it alone, as I did, head to a health food store or baby emporium with a knowledgeable staff and ask for a trusted brand that's easy on the stomach—especially if you're experiencing morning sickness. If you are the researching type, scout out a vitamin that does not exceed 4,000 IU of vitamin A or 500 ug or mcg (aka microgram) of vitamin D, which can be harmful in excessive amounts. Also, make sure it includes the daily doses of vitamins and minerals listed in the chart at right.

Stick to the directions when taking your vitamins; while mistakenly double-dosing on occasion isn't anything to worry about, it's not recommended that you exceed the daily allowance of certain nutrients (especially vitamin A and the aforementioned vitamin D), which in extreme amounts could be harmful to your fetus. Also, skip taking any supplements without your doctor's specific recommendation or approval.

Daily Doses

- At least 400 ug folic acid
- 250 mg (aka milligram) calcium
- 50 mg vitamin C
- 30 mg iron
- 15 mg zinc
- 2 mg vitamin B6
- 2 mg copper
- trace amounts of thiamin, Niacin, vitamin B12, riboflavin, and vitamin E

Check out this chapter's cheat sheet of food no-nos.

This is one instance where you really should not put off until tomorrow what you can do today. Unless you are just finding out you're pregnant six months after conception (you wouldn't be alone; I personally know two mommies who completely missed the first two trimesters), you are in the middle of a very critical time for your embryo's development during which even my wildest mommy-to-be friends put their food and drink intake in check. Read up on the essentials now so you can make educated eating decisions.

If you're taking any prescription

or over-the-counter medications, call your doctor to find out if it's safe to continue. Some pills, liquids, gels, or creams, and even herbal remedies may not be suitable for your developing darling. But if you've been popping pills or gulping cough syrup, don't freak. Instead, give your doctor a ring and find out what's kosher.

Make a doctor's appointment.

Some everyday OB-GYNs won't do the trick since not all of them see moms to term or deliver babies. If yours doesn't, you'll need to hook yourself up now for the next nine months, the big day, and beyond. You should make your first appointment once you realize you are pregnant, although some doctors may not want to see you until eight to ten weeks past the first day of your last period. Check out Chapter 2 for details on how to pick a doctor and other medical minutiae.

Decide when to tell.

Some people choose to keep their swelling status a secret until the three-month mark, when the likelihood of miscarriage is dramatically

> ### Pregnancy on the Sly
>
> One surefire way to tip off your friends to your new and secret status is to suddenly go from a cocktail-wielding party girl to a poster child for sobriety. But you can fake them out at home by sipping pomegranate juice rather than red wine. (Don't refrigerate it or your glass will gather condensation and give you away.) White grape juice can pass for white wine, while cocktails are easily mocked when given the proper glassware and garnish. If you're bar bound, slip the bartender your bottle of juice with a generous tip and instructions to stealthily serve you "the usual" (wink, wink) each time you order. Bottoms up!

lower. Others opt for confiding in only those people that they would turn to for support anyway if things don't work out. Not me. My husband Colie and I agreed to tell only a few select people, but within the first eight weeks we were attending a wedding dinner and I was so loose-lipped I may as well have announced it on stage over the microphone.

Decide, with your partner, who you want to tell.

Personally, I'm not embarrassed to share anything that happens in my life with anyone, and miscarriage—the threat of which causes many women to wait to spill the beans—is a heck of a lot more common than most of us girls know. Just bring it up with friends and you'll be surprised at how many of them will confide that they've had one, or more.

Do what feels right for you, but if you can stomach it, tell at least one mommy girlfriend you are pregnant so that you can complain, wonder, rant, and marvel to someone who is more empathetic and sympathetic than your partner, who's bound to tire of hearing about it even if he or she humors you otherwise.

Also, think carefully about how and when you want to break the news to your boss and coworkers before you let your status slip at the water cooler.

Forget the idea of a "normal" pregnancy.

I don't care what anyone says. There is no such thing as a "normal" pregnancy. Every experience is different, for better and for worse, and even women who've given birth to a large brood will tell you that their experiences have varied dramatically every single time. You may hate being pregnant. You may love it. You may feel like a dead woman walking or more gorgeous and alive than you've ever felt before. You may have every pregnancy ailment known to woman. Common early symptoms can include spotting or having a light menstrual period, feeling like you're going to hurl, breasts that are crazy-tender and swollen, exhaustion, a never-ending need to pee—especially in the middle of the night—moodiness, and general bloating. Or you may have virtually no symptoms at all. Or you may have all of these experiences at different times—perhaps all in the same day. Let the fun begin!

Whatever the case, try not to give yourself a hard time if your adventure doesn't adhere to your expectations or the guidelines set by pregnancy books. Listen to, trust, and care for your body, let it do its thing, and anytime something doesn't feel right, call your practitioner.

Know that fear is natural.

Most mommies-in-waiting experience fear and anxiety for a number of reasons, especially during the first trimester. For most women I know, and for me, our biggest concern was the possibility of losing the baby, a not-so-rare occurrence during the first three months—and sometimes beyond. But before I tail-spun into hormone-heavy tantrums I told myself a few things that may help you, should you fall prey to the worrisome What Ifs.

First, as long as you are taking good care yourself—eating well, drinking water, taking vitamins, resting, skipping pregnancy no-nos (drugs, alcohol, and the special foods outlined in this chapter), and avoiding stress whenever possible—you are doing everything you can to ensure your baby's wellbeing.

Second, if something happens after you've done all of that, it is beyond your control. I firmly believe that if it is the right time for your baby to come into the world, it will, and if it's not, it won't. I have lots of friends who have had multiple miscarriages and who later had happy, healthy babies. You probably also know women who have had such an experience, whether you are aware of it or not. It's a sad fact of life that is unfortunately not openly acknowledged or discussed.

Third, there is nothing more mentally unhealthy and futile than a stressed-out, fatalistic attitude. Besides, if having a baby were that difficult, we wouldn't be struggling with overpopulation!

There are other common fears. On my way to the hospital to give birth I joked, "I was ready to get pregnant, not to have a baby!" I was only half kidding. The unknown can be a very scary concept—especially when you know the coming change is not reversible or temporary and, if you're a first timer, remotely familiar or comprehensible. Lots of women worry about how their lives

> "Listen to your body."
>
> According to the Mommy Menagerie, this was the #1 piece of pregnancy advice to follow.

Want to know when you're due?
Calculate your estimated delivery date by subtracting three months from the first day of your last period. Add a week and there you have it. For example, I last broke out the tampons on November 7 so my due date was August 14.

When's yours? _____

A Few Words on Miscarriage

Here's the dilemma: If I go into miscarriage details I may bum your pregnancy high, but if I don't and you happen to have one, you will really wish you had this information. So here it is.

Don't worry yourself over the possibility—it's a pointless endeavor. And should the stats bring you down, know that 28 of the 30 women mentioned below had successful pregnancies.

Out of 104 mothers who answered the question of miscarriage:

- 33 had confirmed miscarriages.
- 17 out of 33 had 1 miscarriage.
- 12 out of 33 had 2 miscarriages.
- 3 out of 33 had 3 miscarriages.
- 1 out of 33 had more than 4 miscarriages.

Should you have a miscarriage and need emotional support or further information, ask your provider for local sources or search the Internet, where you'll be amazed at the number of support groups and chat rooms.

will change, how their relationships with their partners will change, or whether they will be good mothers.

When you get pangs of fear, acknowledge that it is natural and understandable, give yourself the opportunity to express your feelings to a sympathetic ear or journal (a great way to release tension is to put it on paper), and then, if you can, let them go and instead focus on treating yourself. You now officially have every reason to pamper yourself silly, so why not start immediately!

Go on with your fabulous self!

You're set with the basics and have some time before you head to the doctor. What now? Live your life! Go to work, go out to dinner, see movies, take naps, feel exhausted, cry at cheesy commercials, exercise or don't, admire your soon-to-expand body (and take photos for mementos), dream of your future family, think of baby names, cram yourself into your favorite clothes while you're still able, and enjoy yourself as best you can—even if you have to do it while gagging from morning sickness or tiptoeing around headaches. Soon enough your life will not be your own—seriously—and self-indulgence will be replaced by the rewards, challenges, and relentlessness of parenthood.

This is your time, so make the most of it. Savor every wild and wacky moment and do your best to keep a sense of humor. Trust me: it's your best defense when you are walking down the street, catch a glimpse of your figure in a window, and mistake yourself for a house with legs.

Food No-Nos

Some pregnant women heed all the following food rules, and others risk eating or drinking risky items based on their own comfort levels. As my doctor wisely advised me, make sure that whatever you do won't cause you to blame yourself and your actions should anything go wrong. In other words, if it feels risky, go with your gut and skip it. FYI, if you're looking for more in-depth food facts, you'll find plenty of other tasty tidbits in Chapter 3.

 ### Raw eggs

You're not likely to crave them but they can sneak into your snacks through Caesar salad dressing, cookie dough, cake batter, and half-cooked comforts like eggs Benedict. The danger in raw-egg dining lies in listeria monocytogenes, a bacterium that if present can cause flu-like symptoms in you but create a much worse and possibly fatal scenario in an infected unborn child. The good news is that cases of listeriosis are rare and those that are caught can be treated with medication. Even better is that you can have your cake batter and eat it too if you cook with pasteurized eggs, which are labeled as such on the carton. They eliminate the potential for the food-poisoning-inducing bacteria known as salmonella.

 ### Raw seafood

Sorry, sushi, sashimi, tuna tartare, and oysters on the half shell will have to wait a few more months for the same reasons that raw eggs are not recommended. Another reason to chuck your chopsticks: If not frozen before, raw fish can contain parasites such as tapeworms, which once ingested could grow large enough to steal a good portion of the nutrients meant for your fetus.

 ### Raw or undercooked meat

"I'll have my burger well-done and hockey-puck hard, please." Yup, this is another possible listeria legacy.

 ### Unpasteurized dairy products

Looming listeria strikes again. In case you've been enjoying the liberty, think twice about drinking milk straight from the cow. (Though in truth if you actually went teat-to-mouth the dairy wouldn't have time to tarnish.) Ditto eating raw (unpasteurized) cheeses. Most cheeses sold in the U.S. of A. are pasteurized, but to be sure, read the label on your favorite hunk or ask your local cheese department manager what's off limits.

 ### Soft cheeses

That's right! Due to listeria most medical professionals say brie, blue cheese, camembert, and other deliciously oozy or crumbly dairy delights aren't the pregnant woman's friend. A Parisian girlfriend of mine says even the French are freaked over cheese and unborn bébés. That said, according to the non-profit health biological research foundation Institut Pasteur, France has held steady for the past decade with between 181 and 230 cases of listeria per year, while America's numbers recently suggested that 1 out of about 400,000 people gets infected.

 ### Pâte

Sorry, but this savory spread can also carry listeria.

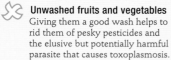

Smoked or processed meats

Any of the above, such as hot dogs, cold cuts, and cured meats, can contain potentional cancer-causing nitrates. Additionally, slabs of luncheon meat sweating behind glass can be lovers for listeria and E. coli—even when refrigerated. Reheating them until they steam ensures safe passage.

Unwashed fruits and vegetables

Giving them a good wash helps to rid them of pesky pesticides and the elusive but potentially harmful parasite that causes toxoplasmosis. (See the cat litter box tip on page 26 for more details.)

Fish high in a form of mercury

Current reports say it's fork off to shark, swordfish, tilefish, and king mackerel, which contain high enough amounts of mercury to possibly harm a fetus's developing nervous system.

More than 12 ounces of fresh fish, shellfish, or canned fish per week

Fish is great for you, but it's recommended you limit portions to manage the inevitable mercury intake. According to the U.S. Department of Health and Human Services, an average of 12 ounces of fish per week is kosher. Some of the safest seafood choices include shrimp, canned light tuna, salmon, pollock, and catfish.

Food prepared on an unwashed surface after contact with raw fish, poultry, or meat

Scrub the heck out of your kitchen counters and cutting boards. If you want to be super safe, put plastic boards in the dishwasher and pop wooden ones in your microwave to kill any possible lingering bacteria.

Drink No-Nos

Alcohol

Some gals, like my French friend and all her mommy pals in Paris, go for the occasional glass of wine, and some doctors give "moderate" consumption the thumbs-up. But if you're a "better safe than sorry" type of girl, it won't kill you to stay dry for the duration. Heavy drinking (multiple indulgences per day) can cause Fetal Alcohol Syndrome, which can result in mental retardation and serious deformities. There is no evidence that the occasional cocktail or glass of wine has similar results, but there is no proof to the contrary either, so medical associations generally discourage the consumption of any alcohol. For the record, I periodically tasted wine (sipped, aerated, and spat) throughout most of my pregnancy. As the person responsible for writing *In Style* magazine's party guides, and recommending wines for each of them, I had to stay on top of the best current-release options. But to be honest, had I wanted the occasional glass of vino, I would have indulged without hesitation. However, even a sip gave indigestion, so the notion never appealed to me.

Excessive caffeine

Refrain from indulging in more than two hot or cold caffeinated drinks per day. While The American College of Obstetricians and Gynecologists says there's no proof that small amounts of caffeine cause pregnancy problems, they also point out that as a stimulant and diuretic, caffeine inspires lots of trips to the ladies room and stops you from snoozing when you need to. By the way, you're not out of the woods if you're not a coffee drinker. You can get just as jacked up on chocolate and many types of soda and tea.

Everyday Activity No-Nos

Are mani-pedis still doable?
You betcha. Add some sparkles to your regular selection for a playful pregnancy pick-me-up.

What about hair dye?
You go on and revitalize your blond, brunette, or black-haired babealiciousness. Today's hair dyes, according to The College of American Obstetricians and Gynecologists, are believed safe for use during pregnancy.

How about squeezing into those tight pants?
Early in the game, it's all good. Soon enough you'll be uncomfortable enough to happily say goodbye to waist-huggers and hello to low- or loose-fitting comfort clothes.

Is it true that saunas and hot tubs are off limits?
Yes, these regularly relaxing spa perks aren't ideal for the new incubating you since they can overheat your body temperature and possibly affect your developing tot.

What about hot baths—with and without bubbles?
The reason hot tubs are on the no-no list is because they can overheat your body and as a result, your growing baby. According to The American College of Obstetricians and Gynecologists, you should not increase your core body temperature above 102.2°F (39°C) for more than 10 minutes or steep yourself to the point that you feel uncomfortable or start sweating. So, go ahead and bob your growing belly in a warm bath and, if there's any question of whether the water is too hot, stick a thermometer in it.

Is the cat litter box another danger zone?
Indeed it is. The fear is around a rare condition called toxoplasmosis, which is introduced by a parasite that can be found in the feces of a cat that has eaten an infected rodent or bird. It can also be found in soils and undercooked contaminated meats. The Center for the Evaluation of Risks to Human Reproduction states that it's a rare occurrence, infecting one to two per one thousand babies born each year in the United States. They also say that if contracted by a pregnant woman, there is a 40% chance that her unborn child will become infected. Regardless, it's a good excuse to get your partner to dig out the dung for a solid nine months, so why not? If you don't have that option, wear gloves when cleaning the box or gardening, steer clear of sandboxes—which cats mistake for backyard bathrooms—and wash your hands thoroughly afterward. Sorry, dog owners, you can still safely scoop your pet's poop.

Is jet-setting still an option?
So long as you have a smooth-sailing pregnancy there's no reason why you shouldn't tote your tummy across the globe if you want. Just remember to bring your medical records in case of an emergency, drink extra water, and stay put after 36 weeks.

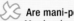

What about exercise?
There are so many answers to this question, and they range from free-for-alls to "absolutely not" depending on whom you ask. But I like the moderate middle's approach, which has recently gained popularity within the medical community: Exercise is GOOD so long as you feel comfortable, never overexert yourself, and do not increase the strenuousness of your regular regime.

(Some doctors also recommend keeping your heart rate below a certain number of beats per minute. Ask your practioner if you're interested in learning more.) Trust your body, use common sense, consider prenatal yoga, and see Chapter 8 for more workout wisdom.

 How about massage? And what's this I hear about the danger of foot massage?

Depends who you ask. Some professionals warn against massage during the first trimester, fearing that it heightens the potential for miscarriage. Others beg to differ, so you really need to go with your gut on this one. Regardless, massage is so beneficial later in pregnancy that it should be a regular right of passage. (The exception is any woman who has a high-risk pregnancy or other pregnancy problems; if that could be you, check with your provider first.) Massage should be scheduled with a trained pregnancy massage therapist who will understand and cater to your sensitivities, including specific acupressure points in the legs, ankles, and feet that correspond to the reproductive system and should be avoided.

 Is sex safe?

About as safe as it's ever going to be, so long as you're monogamous and with a partner you know to be "clean," so to speak. You're already knocked up, so feel free to knock boots. Also, don't be afraid to break out Astroglide or K-Y lubricating jelly. Trust me, you're likely to need it. And don't worry if there's a little bleeding. My doctors said it's normal, so long as it isn't heavy and it dissipates within 48 hours.

Medications Cheat Sheet

The medications listed below were given the a-okay for pregnant women by San Francisco's mommy-mecca California Pacific Medical Center. Be sure to consult your practitioner before popping any other pills, downing any medicinal herbs, prescriptions, or over-the-counter remedies, or slathering on medicinal skin creams. If you're taking medication that was prescribed before you got pregnant, consult your practitioner immediately.

- **Allergies:** Benadryl

- **Congestion:** plain Sudafed

- **Constipation:** Colace or Metamucil

- **Cough:** Robitussin DM

- **Diarrhea:** Kaopectate/Imodium

- **Headache and Fever:** regular strength Tylenol

- **Heartburn:** Gelusil, Mylanta, and Pepcid AC, Tums, and Zantac

- **Yeast Infection:** Gyne-Lotrimin and Monistat

Are You Having a Boy or a Girl?

When I got pregnant I knew I was having a girl from the very first day. It was just a feeling—but one that was so strong that I said to my husband, "How about you pick the boy name and I'll pick the girl name?" Maybe it was a little manipulative, but hey, I could have been wrong. Besides, I'd had our daughter's name selected since I was eight years old. When at 17 weeks we had an ultrasound and learned that we were indeed having a girl, we began calling her by her name, Viva, from that day forward. Had I wagered my child's sex based on the old wives' tales listed below I would have been right—while some "indicators" were off, the majority of them pointed toward a girl. When you've got a few months under your belt, try it and see…

It's a boy if . . .

- When you add your age at the time of conception and the number of the month you conceived, the sum is an even number.

- The dad-to-be is packing on the sympathy weight.

- You skipped morning sickness in early pregnancy.

- Headaches are a regular occurrence.

- You've never looked better!

- You look like you've stuffed a basketball under your shirt.

- Your nose is getting wider.

- Your leg hairs are growing like weeds!

- Your areolas get a serious suntan without sun exposure.

- Your pee is Easter-egg yellow.

- You crave salty or sour foods or proteins.

- Your baby's heart rate doesn't exceed 140 beats per minute.

- Your tootsies are chillier than usual.

- Your hands are as dry as the desert.

- Your bump rides low.

- A ring swings back and forth when dangled from a string over your belly.

It's a girl if . . .

- When you add your age at the time of conception and the number of the month you conceived, the sum is an odd number.

- Your age when you conceived and the year that you conceived are both even or odd numbers.

- Your junk is in the trunk and your hips rather than your tummy area.

- You got intimate with morning sickness during your first trimester.

- PMS is nothing compared to your pregnancy moods.

- Pregnancy doesn't become you.

- You look like you stuffed a watermelon under your shirt.

- You look like you got a boob job.

- Your left breast could beat your right if both were in a wet tee-shirt contest where size mattered.

- Your hair turned slightly redhead.

- Your pee is a dull yellow color.

- Sweets are your craving of choice.

- Your baby's heart rate is at least 140 beats per minute.

- Your face reminisces the breakouts of your teen years.

- You are carrying high.

- A ring swings in a circular motion when dangled from a string over your belly.

When I set out to pick an obstetrician, rather than asking friends or people I trusted who had gone through pregnancy, I got two referrals for doctors who were affiliated at my hospital of choice from the receptionist at my trusted OB-GYN (aka obstetrician-gynecologist). I made appointments to see both, figuring it was worth the price of an extra office visit to have the choice to pick my favorite OB.

But before my first appointment, my OB-GYN recommended another doctor altogether, who, fortunately, was a member of one of the practices I was scheduled to visit. This doctor, she told me, delivered her baby and was great because she had a no-nonsense, relaxed approach to pregnancy—just like me. As I was able to meet her doctor during my upcoming visit to her offices, I kept my other appointments.

Three days before my appointment with the other practice, their receptionist called to tell me my doctor was predisposed and needed to reschedule. I had planned my whole day around the appointment, so I was less than thrilled. But my lack of enthusiasm kicked into alarmingly fierce pregnant-woman rage when I was told the next available appointment was 10 days out. I promptly informed the receptionist that their lame first impression was enough to knock them out of the running.

My next appointment didn't fare much better. I walked in excited, ten weeks pregnant, and anticipating a kind, understanding doctor to lead me and Colie, who had tagged along, through the process. What we got was an ice queen. With nary a "Congratulations!" or "How are you feeling?" she informed us that I currently had a 30% chance of losing the baby, just because that was the average stat before the first ultrasound—which we were about to do in the next minute! When she stuck a condom-covered, vibrator-like ultrasound wand inside me, I tried to lighten the mood by turning to Colie, who sat wide-eyed beside me, and asked, "Jealous?" The queen didn't even crack an ice-smile. Upon hearing our fetus's heart beating for the first time, her warm and fuzzy response was, "Now you're down to the 10th percentile."

Needless to say, I kicked her to the curb—politely, since I was not at that moment in the middle of one of my spontaneous rages—and scheduled my next visit with the doctor recommended by my gyno. Turns out she was a dream. Straightforward but warm, she shared my relaxed views on pregnancy, made Colie and me feel excited to be there, and left us feeling positive every time we walked out the door.

Bedside manner goes a long way during this intimate, thrilling, and sometimes frightening experience. Try to take the time to find someone who makes you feel comfortable—especially when she's inserting a wand up your yoo-hoo.

SORTING OUT THE MEDICAL MINUTIA

Once you discover you're pregnant your doctor may see you to confirm your status with a blood test, but you usually won't begin that oh-so-personal journey with the person who will guide you from inception to delivery until you're eight to ten weeks along. Why? Because that's the time they generally like to do the first exam and give you a vaginal ultrasound—the first of many not-so-modest interactions—and tell you whether you're safely on your way or not. Yes, the days leading up to it can be frustrating and full of anticipation, anxiousness, and impatience. But on the bright side, you can put all of your nervous energy toward setting yourself up with the perfect medical ambassador and palace in which to welcome your baby into the world. In other words, this waiting period is the prime time to get down to the business of picking a birthing facility and delivery doctor, midwife, or whomever else you want to oversee your birth.

Some women follow the prevailing path of using a doctor and giving birth in a hospital. Others go alternative routes with home deliveries and midwives or something in between. Regardless, whether you're in a position to pop bonbons and linger over soap operas all day or barely have time for a bathroom break, you can—and will—benefit from investing time up front in sorting out the medical minutia, making some birthing decisions, and taking the following steps so you can rest assured that you've set yourself up for success. Read on to learn more about your choices and take a peek at this chapter's pregnancy timeline cheat sheets, which will be here for you any time you want to be reminded how far along you and your baby are in the developmental path to family life.

Pick where you'll give birth.

Unless you're considering a home birth or like a particular medical practice enough to follow wherever they lead, you should first determine the hospital or medical facility where you want to perform your grand finale. It sounds ridiculous, but the reason you want to decide this first is because you'll want to choose a doctor who has the authority to deliver at your preferred location. If you've got the time, check out the various local facilities to see what looks the most clean and comfy for you. Or ask around to make sure it has a good rep among your mommy friends and doctors. Other factors to consider include the disposition of the staff, availability of private rooms, showers or bathtubs (good for women going through labor without drugs), statistics on the hospital's percentage of vaginal versus C-section births (especially if you would prefer a vaginal birth), proximity to your residence, and, of course, insurance coverage.

Next, ask your friends,

family, and doctor for good board-certified practitioner referrals.

Get specific about what kind of health provider you prefer. The obstetrician-gynecologist is the most specialized within traditional

Learn More

If any medical advice you receive doesn't sit well with you, don't automatically accept it. Research! Get second opinions! Doctors are not gods. They're people with opinions, attitudes, and preferences, just like everyone else. The more educated you are about your medical options, the more equipped you will be to make educated decisions about your pregnancy and birth, and to verbalize your preferences to professionals.

Who Should Deliver the Goods?

Along with more than one type of place to deliver your baby, there are also various types of specialists to conduct the effort.

Obstetrician = a.k.a. OB-GYN, these women's healthcare specialists have put in an extra four years of study time into women's basic and reproductive issues so they've got all of the fetus and mommy medical issues covered, from the everyday to the specialized stuff. They generally deliver babies within a hospital setting.

Maternal-Fetal Medicine Specialists = The favorite for high-risk pregnancies, these docs have taken studies a step beyond OB-GYNs with two to three years of additional training and certification in the high-risk arena. They also tend to be hospital-centric.

Family physician = The good ol' fashioned family doc has put in three years of overtime in the area of family medicine, which includes obstetrics. Not as specialized as the OB-GYN, this pro can, however, deliver your tot in a hospital and continue to tend to you and your family years after you've forgotten the pangs of labor.

Certified Nurse-Midwife = These alternatives to the status quo are empathetic holistic practitioners who give your emotional, intellectual, and medical needs equal attention and generally help you deliver your dreamboat in a hospital, but also potentially a birthing center or home. Often turned to when there's a strong desire for a drug-free vaginal birth combined with a low-risk pregnancy, these specialists are registered nurses who are licensed and board-certified and have a graduate degree in midwifery. (It's always a good idea to confirm their certification and license within your state.) They also coordinate with qualified doctors if and when backup or support is necessary.

Direct-Entry Midwife = Usually employed by women who prefer a home or pregnancy center birth, these practitioners will walk you down the pregnancy aisle, can help you get necessary tests, and even refer you to a doctor if and when needed. They may or may not be certified through the North American Registry of Midwives (narm.org) and likewise may or may not be covered by your healthcare plan, so if you're thinking of going this route, do some research on both issues and decide if it works for you.

medicine. You can also choose a family practitioner or midwife. In any case, determine if your potential doctor's practices, preferences, and bedside manner fit your ideals beforehand. After all, you don't want to be screaming for an epidural only to discover that your doctor is a fierce proponent of natural childbirth—or, conversely, want to wait out a slowly advancing labor with a doctor who is famed for knee-jerk C-sections. Also, don't be afraid to call and pepper the staff with questions before you even get in the door—and throughout your entire pregnancy, for that matter. They're used to it. And besides, if they don't take the time to appease your fears and qualify themselves, it's a good indication of what kind of treatment you can expect.

Don't forget to make sure your doctor

has access to the hospital you want. If not, determine which is more important to you—the warm and fuzzy doctor with the steady hands or the clean bed with the nice view.

Confirm that your insurance covers your choice.

The price of giving birth can vary from that of a modest American sedan for a vaginal birth to that of a European luxury convertible for a C-section. Considering the costs of decorating your baby's room and stocking up on diapers, baby food, and cute little outfits—never mind raising a child—you will want to squeeze every penny you can.

Research the type of delivery you want to have.

Today's choices make determining what kind of birth you want to have more baffling than your first walk down the diaper aisle at the grocery store. You can go for a home birth with groovy music and meditation; release your tot into a warm water bath; squat, push, and rely on gravity from a birthing chair; or elect for a doctor to pull that baby right out of you without ever opening your legs (aka C-section).

Even if you're predisposed to the standard OB-GYN/hospital/vaginal birth route, you still have decisions to

Mommy Menagerie Fact

88 members of the Mommy Menagerie divulged whether they went with a doctor or a midwife for their combined 94 pregnancies. The results? 80% were delivered by a doc while the other 20% had babies welcomed to the world by a midwife.

"Ask your friends, family, and doctor for good practitioner referrals."

make—including if you want to get doped up the instant you waddle in the door or hold out and try to find peace with the pain. You've got months to conceive of your birthing plan and its nuances so don't start fretting just yet. But it's a good idea to educate yourself earlier in your pregnancy rather than on your way to the delivery room. Take it from someone who knows: If your birth doesn't go the way you wanted it to, you'll feel better knowing that the choices you made when it came down to B-day—and those that you let your practitioner make on your behalf—didn't direct you away from your birthing dreams. That said, when the time comes it may be that nothing works out the way you expected or planned. And there are issues that may change your mind for you at the 11th hour, such as a baby that's not optimally positioned for a trip south or is stressing out about its imminent relocation. In that case, it helps to remind yourself that your number one priority is a healthy baby and mom regardless of how you get there.

Educate yourself on Amniocentesis versus CVS

if you're a candidate. If you're under 35 or have a low-risk pregnancy, you may not be presented with the proposition to undergo an Amniocentesis or Chorionic villus sampling (CVS), two tests that measure your baby's potential for serious genetic disorders, such as sickle cell anemia, Down's syndrome, or hemophilia. But after being subjected to statistics that show how fetus disorders increase with your age, most women 35 and older are faced with the decision of which test to take, if any at all. The decision can be a stressful and fearful one, especially if you don't educate yourself about your options. Along with reading this primer and additional materials, I highly recommend chatting with your provider about your options and asking mommy friends about their experiences.

A CVS procedure involves the withdrawing of a placenta tissue sample through your cervix or your abdomen with a catheter (a thin tube) or a needle. It can be done at around 10 weeks, so it also allows you the opportunity to make serious decisions during your first trimester if something is actually wrong. It becomes less accurate after 13 weeks, which is when you get into amnio territory.

An amnio can be conducted early in your second trimester, at around 16 weeks. The process includes withdrawing amniotic fluid through a sizable needle stuck into your midsection and getting it tested—a notion that naturally fills most soon-to-be mommies with fear. But it is considered the most accurate way to test for disorders.

Pump It Up!
Your body's blood volume increases by 50% during pregnancy!

Both procedures are thought of as a little risky because studies show that women who have undergone these tests have a slightly higher rate of miscarriage.

Some women take the less conclusive and non-invasive nuchal translucency screening between 11 and 14 weeks and/or the AFP multiple marker screening given from around 14 to 20 weeks, before taking an amnio. These tests can offer some clues as to whether you're high risk for a chromosomal problem or really should follow up with an amnio. But they won't leave you without a shadow of a doubt.

Whether you choose to go for any test is a very personal decision that deserves some education and research beforehand—and requires you to consider what you would do if you learned your fetus has a serious disorder. Should you opt for a test you may be counseled beforehand by a genetic counselor that will discuss statistics based on age and your and your partner's ethnicities.

Because I was over 37 and forever the type who likes cold hard facts, I went for the amnio. My plan was to hold, or rather squeeze the life out of, Colie's hand, and look at his face from the time the needle was within blocks of my presence until after it was in the toxic-waste bin. I made him promise not to look at the needle, just in case his eyes bulged like a cartoon character at the sight of the thing—which would certainly have freaked me out. But none of that was necessary.

During the process I felt absolutely nothing, got to find out my baby's sex (they'll ask if you want to know before divulging anything), and witnessed her dancing (pumping her arms and legs) via an ultrasound monitor, which the doctor watches to ensure the needle and baby are nowhere near each other. The weirdest part of the whole experience was the long duration of the procedure; it took what seemed like several minutes to withdraw the fluid.

Still, don't blindly follow my lead. Know what you're getting into. If you're considering one of these tests you can make an educated decision by doing some research online, learning more through your practitioner, or reading books.

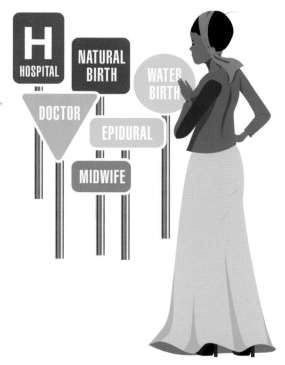

Body Language: Common Pregnancy Peculiarities

Here's a fun list of ways your body may remind you that it's been invaded. Don't be alarmed. As I've said before, you're not likely to experience all of them and, even if you do, it certainly won't happen all at once. Just for fun, check those that apply then flip to Chapter 6 to find out how to get rid of some of them, make others more tolerable, or at least find sympathy and the humor in them.

yep	nope		yep	nope	
☐	☐	Acne	☐	☐	Enlarged vagina
☐	☐	Back soreness	☐	☐	Estrogen spots on arms and chest
☐	☐	Bleeding gums	☐	☐	Exhaustion
☐	☐	Bloating—hands, feet, and everything in between	☐	☐	Faintness, dizziness, or fainting
☐	☐	Bloody noses	☐	☐	Fast hair growth—and not just on your head
☐	☐	Breast pain	☐	☐	Frequent urination
☐	☐	Broken capillaries in face/chest	☐	☐	Food aversions or cravings
☐	☐	Carpal tunnel syndrome	☐	☐	Forgetfulness
☐	☐	Chafing thighs	☐	☐	Gas
☐	☐	Change in sense of balance	☐	☐	Giant (possibly painful) breasts
☐	☐	Chapped lips	☐	☐	Headaches
☐	☐	Constipation	☐	☐	Heartburn/indigestion
☐	☐	Contractions (Braxton-Hicks)	☐	☐	Hemorrhoids or rectal bleeding
☐	☐	Dark line from your crotch to your bellybutton—aka the linea nigre	☐	☐	Hip aches
☐	☐	Darkening of freckles			

yep	nope		yep	nope	
☐	☐	Intensified sense of smell	☐	☐	Rashes
☐	☐	Itching	☐	☐	Reflux
☐	☐	Joint pain	☐	☐	Restless leg syndrome
☐	☐	Larger feet	☐	☐	Shortness of breath
☐	☐	Leaking breasts	☐	☐	Sight loss
☐	☐	Leg cramps	☐	☐	Snoring
☐	☐	Lower back and leg pain (sciatica)	☐	☐	Stretch marks
			☐	☐	Stuffy nose
☐	☐	Moodiness	☐	☐	Swollen hands, ankles, and feet (edema)
☐	☐	Morning sickness			
☐	☐	Mucus increase	☐	☐	Urinary leakage
☐	☐	Nausea	☐	☐	Vaginal discharge
☐	☐	New skin tags	☐	☐	Varicose or spider veins
☐	☐	Nipple size/color change	☐	☐	Yeast infections
☐	☐	Overheating			
☐	☐	Pregnancy mask			
☐	☐	Protruding belly button			

Learn as much as you can

about birthing options before you go into labor! While I imagined holding out on an epidural for as long as possible, going for a vaginal birth, and jovially welcoming my daughter into the world, when my labor hit—and hit hard!—I raced to the hospital and demanded to be admitted. They granted my request only with my consent that they could medically help my progress along.

To make a long story short, I ended up getting enough medication to make me about as mobile and cognitive as a 163-pound anvil; 18 hours later I had a C-section due to a lack of cervical dilation and a stressed-out baby. This path may or may not have been my destiny regardless of whether I blindly agreed to get pumped full of Pitocin and the myriad of other intravenous concoctions that followed. The truth is, I'll never know. But I would have felt much better about the change of course if I had felt confident that my delivery room choices were for good reason and not just because I didn't know any better.

First Doctor's Appointment Cheat Sheet

 Where:
Decide where you want to deliver—hospital, home, Vegas, Namibia, wherever.

 Who:
Pick a doctor or certified nurse-midwife that delivers at your preferred location. Make your first appointment for six to eight weeks after the first day of your last period.

 What:
Ask the doctor's office if they can forward any pregnancy information in advance of your visit.

 When:
Be prepared to inform your doctor about the first day of your last period, any medications you are taking, and the dates of your immunizations, if you can remember them.

 Why:
Keep a list of questions that you want to ask during your appointment and bring it with you. Otherwise, you will forget that you wanted to know whether headaches are normal or if you are doing anything to encourage your new bouts of aches and pains.

 Concerns:
Call your care provider with any concerns—even before your first visit—as many times as necessary.

Expected Tests Cheat Sheet

If you visit the doctor regularly over the course of pregnancy you'll be poked, prodded, pricked, and pried. The following shortlist of tests tells the basics on regularly occurring procedures.

Blood tests:

You are likely to be subjected to a needle in the arm on more than one occasion. The myriad reasons include: determining your blood type; confirming immunity to rubella (German measles) and varicella (chicken pox), which can cause birth defects; testing for infections, such as hepatitis, syphilis, and HIV, anemia, and gestational diabetes; checking if your baby has the potential for fetal defects such as spinal bifida (problems with the neural tube, which becomes the spinal column); and searching for any other medical issues that may need to be treated, monitored, or navigated. It's a piece-of-cake process, provided you aren't the type that passes out at the sight of a needle. (If you are, don't look!)

Urine tests:

You are bound to become quite comfortable toting a tiny jar of urine from the bathroom to the doctor's office. Sometimes taken on the spot and other times conducted as take-home tests, these occur regularly to keep an eye on your body's levels of sugar, protein, and bacteria, which can signal diabetes or bladder or kidney problems. If you're going the take-home route and are still half asleep when you tinkle each morning, put the jar on the toilet seat the night before your doctor visit to ensure you gather the first pee of the day, which is preferred.

Pap tests:

This collection of your cervical secretions can show telltale signs of cervical cancer and other cell abnormalities. It's no different than the mildly uncomfortable poke you receive during your annual checkup. There are an array of other reasons your practitioner takes cultures from your now spotlighted yoo-hoo, including keeping a lookout for HPV (genital warts) and a GBS infection (aka group B streptococcus—a bacteria that's generally harmless to adults and hosted by many women, myself included), which can be passed to the baby during delivery. If you've got 'em, your practitioner will help make sure you don't flaunt 'em.

Glucose Challenge test (GCT):

Well into your incubation period you'll be asked to down a small bottle of supersweet liquid, wait an hour, and then get a blood test to see your body's reaction to being slammed with sugar. The purpose is to diagnose whether you have gestational diabetes, a commonly occurring condition that is specific to pregnant women, easily navigated once diagnosed, and generally naturally resolved shortly after giving birth.

Baby Growth Cheat Sheet

What's going on in there? Plenty, from the minute your egg and that champion swimmer sperm had their momentous rendezvous. Browse this month-by-month meandering of how your baby sprouts from a zygote that's smaller than a pinhead to a full-fledged bundle of joy.

FIRST TRIMESTER (Weeks 1–13)

First Month: The Beat Goes On!

Is that a pinhead in your uterus or are you just happy to see me? Actually, it is a tiny embryo that, at the beginning of the month, floats around and by mid-month attaches to the uterine wall. Its sex has been determined since fertilization. Growth highlights include the beginnings of limb buds—which become arms and legs—the heart, lungs, and neural tube (later to become the brain and spinal cord). By day 22, there's a heartbeat, but it is only audible perhaps to any nearby Whos from Whoville. At the end of the fourth week, your embryo is the size of a grain of rice—about ¼ inch long.

Second Month: Fingers and Toes!

All major body organs and systems are accounted for but still developing in your embryo. Your body has furnished it with a full-service studio apartment complete with plumbing and heating: the placenta. Your little embryo's skeleton is formed. His head and face are taking shape, his umbilical cord has developed, and blood is flowing through his very basic circulatory system. By midmonth it's possible for an ultrasound to pick up his heartbeat. By the end of the month, he has ears, ankles, toes, wrists, fingers, and eyelids that are sealed shut—for now. He's not much longer than the head of a toothbrush—around an inch in length—and at less than 1/3 ounce, he's lighter than a clay poker chip.

Third Month: You've Got Nail!

Your baby can officially be called a fetus from eight weeks onward. Were you a full-service spa, she could request a rudimentary mini mani/pedi this month, as your growing girl has formed soft itty-bitty nails on her fingers and toes. She's also hatched tiny hairs on her newly formed skin and buds in her mouth, which are destined to become baby teeth. Toward the end of the month she can—and will—pee, make a fist, and swallow. Now weighing in at a whopping 1 ounce, she's as tall as a house key or about 2½ to 3 inches long.

SECOND TRIMESTER (Weeks 14-26)

Fourth Month: Busting a Move!

What's your baby up to this month? He's turning his head and kicking and moving like he's on a chorus line. All of his organs and systems are working, so he's now focused on growing, which may explain why you're going to expand at lightning speed too. Just how fast is he sprouting? At the end of the month, were he standing upright on your desk, he'd be a bit shorter than the narrower side of a standard piece of paper, about 6 to 7 inches long, and he'd tip the scale at about 4 to 5 ounces, which is about the same as a cup of hazelnuts. Watch your language! By the 15th week he can hear your voice.

Fifth Month: Innocent Until Proven Guilty!
Good thing you've got a nice baby, because this month were she to get into trouble with the law she could be fingerprinted. Along with developing finger and toe prints, your little one is now getting comfy in her surroundings, taking lots of catnaps, and getting a little exercise by turning sideways and doing summersaults. She can feel touch, can hear better now, and could get startled if you yell, "Boo!" She's a strapping 10 inches in length—just a little longer than a standard-size envelope—and has grown to a hearty ½ to 1 pound.

Sixth Month: Hey! It's Dark in Here!
With red, pruned skin that's coated with soft hair and a waxy substance called "vernix" (it dissolves before his debut), your baby probably couldn't win any beauty contests today, even if he is growing cute little eyebrows and lashes. Although he can now open his eyes and blink, there are no mirrors in your uterus so he's not likely to be self-conscious about his in utero resemblance to An American Werewolf in London. Given his new size—and ever-strengthening bones—a standard piece of paper has nothing on him. At a foot long, he towers a half inch over it, and as a natural pre-born bruiser he is now weighing in at 1½ pounds. Don't hurt his feelings, but do promise him the world; he can cry and dream now, too.

THIRD TRIMESTER (Weeks 27–40)

Seventh Month: No More Barry Manilow, Please!
Your developing bundle of joy is busy this month. He can respond to sound and light, so let him rock out to classical, hip hop, or oldies and don't be surprised if he makes a move when your bulging belly is exposed to bright light. He can pop his thumb in his mouth with ease and stretches and kicks like a yoga-loving soccer player. At 15 to 16 inches, the apple of your abdomen is now tall enough to see eye-to-eye with a Chihuahua, and at 2½ to 3 pounds he might just outweigh it. Now that he's essentially fully formed, he can focus on gaining weight, about a half pound a week until the 37th week. He should also be moving about 10 times per hour. (If he loses momentum, chat with your doctor as soon as possible.) Additionally, your boy is getting clever! Brain development is speeding up now.

Eighth Month: Close Quarters!
If your baby could talk to you, she might say, "You think you feel uncomfortable? Try being balled up inside a bag with no room for a good, hearty stretch, never mind putting your feet up!" But actually, she's comfy in her one-room shack, though she's getting too large to do much else than kick and roll. She's now around 18 inches long and somewhere between 4 and 5 pounds, and has almost fully developed lungs. And she's getting ready for her close-up by beginning to shed her furry, waxy coat.

Ninth Month: Lookout, Mama, Here I Come!
This month your fabulous fetus officially reaches full-term status, complete with lungs that are mature enough not only to function, but also to greet you and the world with a rebel yell that would make Billy Idol proud. If she's mischievous she may be playing hopscotch on your bladder while she continues to gain weight and momentum—ideally by being helpful and dropping into a head-down, ready-for-takeoff position. At 19 to 21 inches and anywhere from 6 to 9 pounds, she's quickly outgrowing her placental palace and is planning to check out soon, leaving you to pay the bill and clean up the mess, thank you very much.

Your Body in Bloom Cheat Sheet

Feel like a walking science experiment yet? If not, you will. Read on to discover all the wacky developmental wonders percolating inside your pregnant body over the next nine-plus months. Don't worry if your pregnancy path doesn't follow suit. Everyone's experience is different.

FIRST TRIMESTER (Weeks 1–13)

First Month: Boil, Boil, Toil, and Trouble

The witches' brew worth of hormones being created and stirred up inside you may come with a curse of extremely tender and swollen breasts, exhaustion, morning sickness, and food cravings. Brace yourself, sister. You ain't seen nothing yet.

Second Month: "I've Gotta Pee!"

Even if you can't tell your body's working, it is! By the fifth week it's already built up a nice protective mucus plug in your cervical canal to ensure your placenta is a private residence for your growing embryo. If it hasn't started already, now's also the time that the pregnancy hormones let your bladder know who's boss by inspiring frequent dashes to the bathroom. Your sore breasts may continue to balloon, while your nipples and areolas could look like they've independently made a few trips to the tanning salon. If you think your midsection seems to be growing in all directions, you are not imagining things. It's making space for your new roommate. Nine weeks into your pregnancy your uterus is the size of a grapefruit. If you're feeling sick and tired, give yourself extra beauty rest.

Third Month: Calgon, Take Me Away!

If you have had it with being exhausted and queasy and you're lucky, at the end of this month you may start feeling superhuman, at least in your energy level. Beforehand you might experience headaches, lightheadedness, dizziness, and wild mood swings—which may or may not have started long before now. Toward the middle of the month your body's continually increasing blood supply partially contributes to that pregnancy "glow." The other factor, pregnancy hormones, can also be responsible for bouts of acne that you haven't experienced since high school.

SECOND TRIMESTER (Weeks 14–26)

Fourth Month: Get a Kick Out of This

This month (and as early as last week) you may receive a distinctive affirmation that some-one has indeed invaded your body—in the form of a flutter, poke, or full-blown kick. Don't worry if your baby hasn't announced his presence. He'll probably make up for it next month by giving you a good ribbing! Meanwhile, if your boobs have been headed toward Pamela Anderson territory, they're not going to stop now, so brace yourself—and if you haven't already, get good support.

Fifth Month: Dance to Your Own Beat

This month or next, depending on your growth, the skin on your belly may begin to itch because your skin is expanding. Your nipples should be growing to become a bulls-eye for a hungry baby—and perhaps a lascivious romantic partner. Even if you are lolling about doing a lot of nothing your heartbeat will increase to help pump more blood to the uterus. You may also get a backache, leg cramps, a lovely patch or two of varicose veins on your legs, or all three ailments. Then there's the ongoing need to pee all the time and that pesky heartburn. Are we having fun yet?

Sixth Month: What Took Over My Body?

Your back may hurt, and your uterus may be stretching enough to make its supporting ligaments feel sore. After standing a good while you may be sporting a new set of cankles—that beautiful transformation that happens when your ankles swell to the same widths as your calves. If you haven't guessed, now may not be the best time to sport skirts.

THIRD TRIMESTER (Weeks 27–40)

Seventh Month: The Final Stretch—Pun Intended

Yes, you are entering stretch-mark territory, and may start seeing them now or later if your family is predisposed to them (if they're not, you are likely to get relatively unscathed). If you're getting Braxton-Hicks contractions—innocent, painless, false-labor reminders of the labor fun to come—it's all good unless you have more than five per hour. If that happens, give your doctor a jingle. In case that's not enough of a rollicking ride for you, say hello to possible constipation, plus loss of balance due to your newly rotund reality.

Eighth Month: Yo Ho Ho and a Bottle of Colostrum

Should your breasts leak this month, it won't be a bottle's worth, but you may spot a few drops of colostrum sneaking out of your nipples. You may also feel stronger contractions or have none at all. By the way, it's not the anticipation of motherhood that's got you breathless. Your body is temporarily using oxygen and carbon dioxide differently right now, forcing increased and shallower respiration, and your crowded diaphragm is sharing breathing space with your baby-to-be.

Ninth Month: Hey Hot Mama!

Used to have an "inny" belly button? Don't be alarmed if it becomes your tummy's distinctly protruding doorbell. It's just a reminder that your special someone will be paying you a visit very soon. Also welcome more swelling to your lower extremities and anticipate that your cervix may begin to dilate and thin (aka efface) for a more accommodating exit for your fully developed baby.

If you're seeking a prenatal-diet role model, don't look to me. Before I was pregnant I was the kind of girl who generally ate very well. I regularly cooked with organic ingredients, steered clear of processed foods, stuck with a mostly wheat-flour-free regime due to an allergic reaction to the stuff, and indulged modestly by finishing the day with a bowl of Häagan Dazs ice cream. But the minute I became a walking incubator, my willpower went out the window with tampons and birth control. I feasted on what I wanted whenever I wanted, was drawn toward junk food and wheat like never before (I ignored my allergies), and ended up practically wiping the cake crumbs off of my face with pregnancy book pages that discussed the "make every bite count" theory.

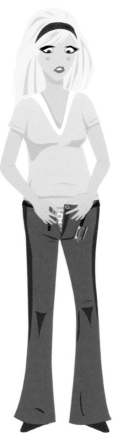

When pregnancy books suggested that I gain between 25 and 35 pounds over the whole duration, I reflected on my many mommy friends who packed on double those amounts and lived to slip back into their pre-pregnancy clothes. So I gave myself a generous top-out weight goal of 35 pounds and abided by a simple rule: eat whatever appeals to me whenever I'm hungry—with the exception of the handful of pregnancy no-nos (I didn't abide by all of them; I ate sushi and sipped wine on occasion).

Often I ate very healthfully—broiled chicken, sautéed vegetables, and my favorite pregnancy salad, (see page 61). But other times it was at least 12 Oreos with two tall glasses of milk in one sitting. As the indulgence menu mounted, I reasoned that devouring a trough of chicken enchiladas or a few handfuls of Cheetos didn't block the benefits of the broccoli and the other very healthful food I was eating; it just added a little more cottage cheese to my quickly expanding thighs.

And boy was I right. I passed the magic weight-gain number at 33-1/2 weeks—and ultimately headed for the delivery room towing an extra 41 pounds. But

I didn't feel badly about it. I reveled in the notion that for the first and only time in my life I was supposed to gain weight. I reasoned that my body was telling me what it wanted and, as a good mother, it was my job to respond. I was probably fooling myself as I imagined my daughter begging for a uterine delivery of chocolate cake and milk. But the truth is, I simply couldn't help myself. I felt a little better knowing that despite doubling up on dessert I still ate a lot of the good stuff and waited for that promised day when the baby would be so big I'd permanently feel "full" for the rest of the pregnancy. Unfortunately, that day never came.

Looking back, I know that some of my cravings were very real and undeniable. But other factors that contributed to my diet were convenience and comfort. Whenever split-second starvation descended upon me and a meal was not within arm's reach, I did not think to stop by a health food store and get nourished on beet salad, grilled tofu, and quinoa. I dashed, mouth agape, toward my favorite comfort foods. Thankfully, stocking up on healthy snacks and bringing my lunch wherever I went stopped me from making a habit of desperation dining.

Do I wish that I had eaten with more restraint? Absolutely. Am I kicking myself for it now? Not at all. I had a healthy, seven-pound, three-and-a-half ounce girl, and a year and a half, a couple of cleanses, and many yoga classes later, I am four pounds away from my pre-pregnancy weight. If I were to do it all again, I'd like to think that I would limit my indulgences and look as fabulous as those celebrity moms parading around in slinky dresses five seconds before—and after—they push out a golden child. But who am I kidding? First off, I didn't look like a superstar to begin with. Secondly, I'm betting I'd mainline Oreos all over again, and at the end of the day I can live with that.

I'm not recommending you use my convenient rationale to have your way with a whole sheet cake. But if you do find yourself uncontrollably shoveling in your favorite snacks, at least you'll know you are in good company.

Whatever the case, remember this: What you put in your body right now directly affects the growth and health of your fetus, so good nutrition is critical. But just as essential is that if and when you fall prey to the seduction of ridiculous treats, you give yourself some slack and go on with your fabulously fattened and satisfied self.

Thought For Food

Food takes on a whole new meaning to the pregnant woman. For some, cravings can result in quests of biblical proportions; I have one friend who made a three-hour round trip just for a specific brand of fresh salsa. For others, especially women experiencing nausea, edibles are dreadful conduits to nutrition that come up with more ease than they go down. And then there's the dilemma of weight gain—an activity that has such a stigma among women in this country that it can be very hard to see yourself as hot *and* heavy.

I'm not going to lie to you. What you put in your body right now matters not only for the health of you and your growing tot, it will also help determine exactly how hard it will be to lose your baby weight afterward. But if you ask me, a lot of the material out there about how we should eat while pregnant is enough to make any mommy who munches on the occasional candy bar feel like she's committed a fetal-related felony.

> "What you put in your body right now directly affects the growth and health of your fetus, so good nutrition is critical."

If you are the type who feels most comfortable following a strict dietary regime and monitoring every morsel, good for you, but unfortunately, you won't find bite-by-bite direction here. (Though you can find online and print sources on page 238.) This chapter isn't going to give you a guilt trip about what you should and shouldn't eat. It will, however, give you the basic guidelines, tips and facts, a hearty dollop of sympathy, and some tasty cravings recipes. Eat up the details here and you can make informed decisions, go about your daily business, and rest assured that you're taking good care of your baby even if the only thing you can hold down on a particular day is a burrito from Taco Bell. Besides, there's no reason to sweat your swelling: If you're becoming Violet Beaurigard minus the blueberry hue, your practitioner will let you know.

Try to eat a well-balanced diet.

In a perfect pregnancy world, the ideal diet is a healthy, well-rounded one. In reality—due to cravings, aversions, nausea, or the sudden need to devour the nearest edible object lest you start gnawing on your office chair—you may not have the luxury of practicing pristine eating habits all the time. Still, even if you partake in lots of pecan pie it's a good idea to embellish it with more healthful stuff, specifically organic fruits, vegetables, whole grains, good carbohydrates, meat, fish, and chicken, or vegetarian protein alternatives.

Keep in mind that you are not really eating for two.

Common consensus is that if you're carrying a single tot you really don't need more than 300 extra calories per day—and that's only if you were consuming a moderate 2,200 calories daily beforehand. So when you head to the fridge remind yourself that "servings" does not mean a heaping Fred Flintstone-size helping. One portion equals about as much as you could palm in your hand—one apple, 1/2 cup of broccoli, one cup of yogurt, two eggs…you get the idea. You could cheat and use Shaquille O'Neal's palm as a barometer, but the only one you'll be fooling is yourself.

Take prenatal vitamins.

If you are healthy and maintain a good diet, your baby is likely to get all of the nutrients he or she needs. But these hefty horse pills are your safeguards. Designed to pick up any nutritional slack, they made me feel like I was taking care of business even on the rare days that I slammed a 10-pack of chicken nuggets and a large fries on my way home from work. Should you be too nauseous to keep these pills down, your doctor can offer advice on navigating the nutrients you need. For the details on the what, where, and why of prenatal vitamins, see page 20 in Chapter 1.

Drink water regularly.

Nothing wilts the pregnant flower like a lack of water. Drink at least 8 glasses a day at a minimum, but shoot for 12.

Know which foods

are no-nos for pregnant women. You can, and should, devour the Food and Drink No-Nos lists on pages 24–25. They include explanations of why a number of everyday foods are not recommended for pregnant women.

Savor Your Splurges

If you're going to splurge on a treat, enjoy it wholeheartedly. While I can completely relate to the guilt associated with overindulging, I believe that if you're going to chow down on something superfluous, the least you can do is savor every bit of it. If your splurges result in misery rather than satisfaction, what's the point? If you give yourself permission to indulge, you should also give yourself permission to feel good about it. Of course this tactic only works if your indulgences are occasional.

Pregnancy by the Pound

Doctors generally recommend that a person of "normal" weight range for their height gain between 25 and 35 pounds. They hike that number by 5 pounds or so for underweight women and decrease it by around 10 pounds for femmes already toting a heavy load. If you're not sure how much you're supposed to gain and you care to know, ask your practitioner. (For the record, I think some perceptions of "normal" are a lot of hooey. At 5 foot, 2 inches, and 122 pounds, I was deemed by an Institute of Medicine of the National Academies chart as weighing in on the high side of normal and a few pounds away from obese—and I had not a pinch of fat on me and wore a size 2 to 4. Give me a break.)

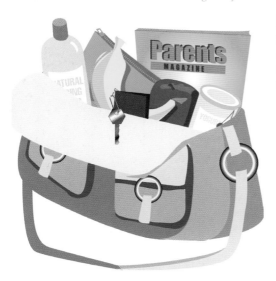

Eat smaller meals

more often. A great way to keep the stomach satisfied early in the game, and avoid indigestion later on, is to snack on six small meals throughout the day rather than eating three big ones.

Limit your intake of stuff

that isn't good for you. The foods and beverages that weren't good for you before pregnancy aren't any better now, and since you're officially force-feeding your unborn babe, you should think twice about trashing his tummy without his consent. In other words, go light on the usual edible foes: refined sugar, processed foods, hydrogenated fats, artificial colors and flavors, foods with preservatives, artificial sweeteners, sodas made with fructose, caffeine, and alcohol.

If you don't want to eat junk,

don't keep it around. I tended to eat very well at home. Although I continued my pre-pregnancy nightly bowl of ice cream early on, it was easy to stop indulging the minute I stopped buying it. For me, out of sight really was out of mind. But beyond the house was a different story. I never bought and rarely ate cookies before, during, or after my pregnancy. But while in waiting, a delivery truck pulled up to my dot-com office once a week and offloaded enough snack food to keep a staff of 20 workaholics hopped up on sugar. While I occasionally reached into the cupboard for a breakfast bar or handful of cashews (or 10), I was more regularly wooed by my nutritional nemesis, the sweets drawer. Stuffed with those aforementioned Oreos and bags of mini Chips Ahoys, it serenaded me regularly and I an-

"A great way to keep the stomach satisfied is to snack on six small meals throughout the day."

What's All That Weight?

Comedian Jenny McCarthy joked that when she went to the hospital to give birth, she was hoping to discover that she was carrying a 60-pound baby. Of course she wasn't. In actuality, the average extra poundage breaks down something like this: 7-1/2 pounds of baby, 1-1/2 pounds of placenta, 2 pounds amniotic fluid, 2 pounds new breast tissue (more if you're like me), 2 pounds uterus expansion, 4 pounds extra blood, and 4 pounds other fluids. The rest is fat stores, which are important and necessary—in moderation—and ideally total between 7 and 12 pounds.

swered its call at least once a week. If you have a similarly sweet work environment and the ability to easily fall from nutritional grace, my recommendation is don't allow yourself to indulge in the free office bootie even once. The minute you cross over to the dietary dark side, it's hard to go back.

Bring food with you

everywhere you go. Packing a picnic of healthy, ever-ready snacks and carrying backups in your purse and car works wonders. When sudden starvation hits, it's the difference between immediate guiltless satisfaction and a carelessly caloric dash for the nearest drive-thru. For a list of easy edibles, see page 54. And don't forget to tote a couple of bottles of water.

Online Sources
Want to learn more about no-no foods? Food phobes will frolic with the jubilance of hippies at a Grateful Dead concert if they browse the facts found on the websites of the Center for Disease Control (www.cdc.gov) and Center for Science in the Public Interest (www.cspinet.org).

Eat good-mood food.

If you're feeling extra cranky or exhausted, take a mental inventory of what you've been eating and consider redirecting your diet. Perhaps eating smaller, more frequent meals will boost your energy or settle your tummy. Maybe you're not eating enough—that'll tire you out, too. Or perchance you're overindulging in sugar or caffeine, which can make a grown adult crash and burn as dramatically as a child who's coming down off of a major ice cream high.

See the Home Remedies chapter

if you need help with nausea. Some bouts of nausea cannot be contained by food alone, but many of them can be calmed with a little dietary forethought. You'll find a feast of tummy-soothing ideas on page 102.

Consider a diet that avoids

heartburn and indigestion. The slowing of digestion that happens during pregnancy doesn't just result in the occasional toot. It also impedes the effectiveness of the valve that connects your stomach with your esophagus, sometimes

Mommy Menagerie's Top 10 Cravings

1. Fruit. 9% had a hankering for fruit, while 30% got particular. In order of popularity: watermelon, oranges, grapefruit, citrus, strawberries, bananas, apples, lemons, pineapple, avocado, blueberries, cantaloupe, peaches, and nectarines.

2. Ice Cream. 18% put this high on their lists, be it served in a bowl, devoured as a sandwich, or spooned straight from the tub.

3. Chocolate. While 5% called for straight-up chocolate, other mommies were lulled by chocolate cake, pudding, cupcakes, and cookies, bringing the calling for cocoa to a solid 10%.

4. Hamburgers or Cheeseburgers. 9%—including one vegetarian—begged for burgers.

5. Cheese. 7% said cheese on a regular basis.

6. A tie between **Taco Bell** and **Red Meat.** A solid 6% put this Mexican fast-food stop or red meat on their list.

7. A tie between **Salad, Lemonade, Root Beer,** and **Coke** (Diet and Regular). 5% looked to bowls of leafy greens, refreshing lemonade, or the bubbliness of root beer or Coke to soothe their souls.

8. A tie between **Eggs, Yogurt, Pickles, Orange Juice,** and **Beer** (alcoholic and non-alcoholic) showed up with 4% of the vote.

9. A tie between **Sushi, Pizza, Cake, Cookies, Milk, Wine, Milkshakes,** and **Macaroni and Cheese** made the list at 3% each.

10. A tie between **Donuts, Apple Pie, Cottage Cheese, Mexican Food, Chocolate Milk, Peanut Butter,** and **Tomatoes** came in at 2% each.

resulting in food moving backward, or coming back up into your esophagus, after it's already made a pass-through and been mingling with gastric acids. When this acidic version of lunch makes its way back upward, it results in heartburn. You may not be able to resolve it completely, but the key is to monitor your body's reactions to the foods you eat and adjust your diet for optimum comfort. For details on how to manage the madness, see Chapter 6, page 98.

Prenatal vitamins have your nutritional back, but certain foods help you face good mommy and baby nutrition head on. Scan the cheat sheet of essentials starting on the next page and see why they're worthy in general and especially essential during certain trimesters, then—rather than obsessing about health—you can confidently munch on foods that deliver the gestational goods.

Food & Drink 10 Commandments

1. Aim for nutrients-rich foods

2. Stay hydrated

3. Take prenatal vitamins

4. Keep healthy snacks around at all times

5. Don't let yourself get too hungry

6. Eat many small portions daily

7. Give in to your cravings, within reason

8. Never try to lose weight

9. Avoid foods that could carry bacteria (see page 24)

10. Don't booze it up or pop any unauthorized pills

Essential Eats Cheat Sheet

 FIRST TRIMESTER

Folic Acid. One of the absolute must-haves, especially during the first trimester, this B vitamin is critical for neural development. Deficiencies are associated with neural tube defects—which result in the most serious and common birth defects. The good news is you can easily get your fill by snacking on leafy vegetables, citrus fruits, beans, some cereals, and whole grains.

Magnesium. Good for developing organs and bones and your own body tissues, this natural metal is also used to help prevent preterm delivery in women with preterm contractions. Serious deficiencies may cause trouble, including kidney problems. So live it up with likeable foods like whole wheat breads, bran muffins, multigrain cereal, broccoli, chard, spinach, sea bass, beans, soy, and nuts.

Potassium. This mineral helps your cells maintain fluid and electrolyte balance, boosts your body's ability to make the most of metabolism, and aids in the transition of nerve impulses. It's also abundant in the average diet. But women with projectile morning sickness should make an effort to increase intake since potassium is also easily depleted. To load up, choke down bananas, strawberries, watermelon, oranges, cantaloupe, raisins, prunes, apricots, dates, beets, spinach, peas, tomatoes, beans, turkey, beef, and grapefruit or prune juice.

Vitamin A. Outstanding for your fetus's cell and tissue growth and eye, ear, limb, and membrane development, this healthy helper will also aid you with postpartum tissue repair. But here too much of a good thing definitely isn't a good thing. In excessive amounts, vitamin A can cause birth defects and liver toxicity. Fortunately, ODing is only a threat if you take it in the form of a supplement or a drug or a skin cream that contains it, such as Retin-A. Get your fill by feasting on dairy, fish, meat, fortified cereals, and fruits and veggies that contain beta-carotene, which converts to vitamin A in your body.

Vitamin B6. This vitamin is known to be an effective therapy for the nauseous mommy-to-be. But more importantly, it helps metabolize protein, aids in your blood cell and antibody production, and works wonders on your fetus's brain and nervous system development. If you needed a good reason to make the Avocado Cream Pie recipe on page 63 now you've got it: Good bets for this vibrant vitamin are avocados as well as bananas, watermelon, potatoes, wheat bran, wheat germ, beef, poultry, and brown rice.

Zinc. This magnificent mineral is crucial for DNA synthesis, a friend to the immune system, and nearly effortless to obtain, especially if you're popping prenatal vitamins. But there are other ways to think zinc, specifically red meat, poultry, beans, nuts, whole grains, fortified breakfast cereals, and pumpkin and sunflower seeds. FYI: Consuming dairy products increases zinc absorption.

SECOND TRIMESTER

Chromium. Marvelous for regulating your blood sugar, this mineral also helps baby's tissues create pertinent protein. Down it in the form of beef, cheese, whole grain bread, apples, eggs, spinach, and oranges.

Iron. As a participant in maintaining a healthy placenta, a building block for red blood cells, and an aid in internal oxygen distribution, this mineral is crucial for your increased blood volume and for the baby who begins storing iron this trimester. You can load up by chowing down on the likes of red meat, the dark meat of turkey and chicken, shellfish, sardines, beans, beets, and spinach.

Potassium. Same drill as above, different trimester.

Protein. This dietary power player and proponent of the healthy placenta is critical throughout pregnancy, especially from your second trimester on when it pumps up cell growth and expanding tissues for you and your little one. It's also said to quell nausea. Find it in milk, yogurt, cheese, cottage cheese, eggs, beans, fish, shellfish, poultry, meat, nuts, and even peanut butter!

Vitamin C. Vital for production of collagen, a component that binds together skin, blood vessels, nerves, and muscles, this vitamin is key in tissue repair, delivery recovery, fighting infection, and building the immune system. Find this healthy-body helper in juicy fruits and lots of vegetables, including oranges, grapefruit, tomatoes, and broccoli.

 THIRD TRIMESTER

Calcium. Give strength to your and your baby's bones, teeth, muscles, and nerves by loading up on calcium-rich foods. Dairy is a good distributor, as are almonds, rice, broccoli, kale, olives, and fortified juices.

Iron. Keep pumping it in, just like last trimester. It'll help you handle blood loss from delivery.

Omega-3 Fatty Acids. Naturally abundant in flaxseeds, walnuts, salmon, and soy beans, these fatty acids are crucial on so many levels. They are imperative for brain development during pregnancy and the first two years of life, have been said to help increase breast milk production, and are reputed to help with heart disease and inflammation. Deficiencies can impede your fetus's nervous and immune systems from fully developing. So, if you can't stomach the foods above, consider sprinkling your waffles or breakfast bread with flaxseed oil, as I do for my daughter every morning.

Protein. That baby's still growing, so on protein, keep mowing.

Vitamin A. Revisit the reasons noted above under the First Trimester essentials. It's also terrific for tissue repair.

Vitamin B6. Consult those First Trimester notes again.

Vitamin C. Ditto.

Zinc. Along with brain development as mentioned at left, zinc helps expedite healing and thus recovery from childbirth.

Snacks Cheat Sheet

When pregnancy hunger hit I was so overwhelmed I found it impossible to muster enough sanity to speak, never mind think logically about what I could eat and where I could find it. So not to suffer the same fate, consider stocking up on snacks, such as the following favorites of the Mommy Menagerie.

1. Breakfast Bars
Belly bars
Clif bars
Fruit & Nut bars
granola bars
Harvest bars
Kashi granola bars
Luna bars
Mojo bars
Zone bars

2. Cereal
Oatmeal (instant)
Teddy Grahams
Cheerios

3. Cheese
cheddar cheese
Jarlsberg cheese
Kraft American Singles
Monterey Jack cheese
string cheese

4. Chips
Baked Lays
potato chips
tortilla chips

5. Crackers and Bread
bread
Goldfish crackers
graham crackers
oyster crackers
peanut butter and cheese
  crackers
pretzels
rice cakes
rice crackers
Ritz crackers
Saltines
stone-ground wheat
  crackers
water crackers
Wheat Thins

6. Dairy
cottage cheese
hard-boiled eggs
ice cream
yogurt

7. Fruit
apples
bananas
dried fruit
grapes
oranges
pineapple
raisins
watermelon

8. Nuts
almonds
cashews
mixed nuts
peanuts
sunflower seeds
tamari almonds

9. Veggies
broccoli florets
carrots
cucumber
edamame
pickles

10. Chocolate
chocolate bars
dark chocolate

11. Candy
"Preggie Pops" lollipops
Devil Dogs
ginger candy
gummy bears
Jolly Ranchers
mints
spearmint gum

12. Spreads & Dips
hummus (with carrot or celery sticks)
peanut butter (with apple slices or crackers)
salsa (mild)
soy butter

13. Other Savory Stuff
frozen waffles
popcorn
soups
trail mix

14. Other Sweet Treats
7-Up
caramel sauce (for dipping apple slices)
cookies
fruit cups
ice cream
ice cream sandwiches
popsicles
Pop-Tarts or organic toaster pastries
sorbet

What Do You Crave?

During my triple-trimester adventure I had newfound love affairs with American cheese, those dreaded Oreos, grapefruit juice, cashews, root beer, ice water (which I previously preferred at room temperature), caviar (alas! this is a no-no food, and yes, I did eat it on occasion, as well as sushi and medium-rare hamburgers), and grilled chicken salad with mango, avocado, and spiced pecans (get the recipe on page 61). I also yearned for but did not partake in margaritas. Pre-pregnancy preferences for chicken tacos and ice cream quickly fell out of favor until after my daughter was born. What are your food faves and foes? Make a list of your cravings and aversions, just for fun.

Love it!

_____
_____
_____
_____
_____
_____
_____
_____
_____

Hate it!

_____
_____
_____
_____
_____
_____
_____
_____

CRAVING RECIPES

The recipes I found in pregnancy books didn't inspire me. I figure most women, like me, know their preferred preparations for healthy foods and aren't about to race to the kitchen to try a recipe for a chickpea and nut loaf. More interesting to me were craving recipes—unabashed celebrations of the whims of the prenatal palate. So, I put out calls to friends who are chefs and parents and asked them to fork over their favorite pregnancy culinary creations. Without further adieu, read on for the tastiest submissions. Some are virtually guiltless indulgences, others are shameless special-occasion treats, but all are downright delicious and easy to prepare.

Chestnut and Celery Soup

My regular job, besides being a mommy, is as a food, wine, and travel writer and entertaining expert. It's a wonderful career that allows me to meet all kinds of incredible people, including executive chef Bertrand Bouquin, who was orchestrating outstanding food at Colorado's Broadmoor resort while I was reviewing it for a magazine. Bouquin trained with many of the world's best chefs before becoming a stud in his own right. But more importantly, he's a loving husband and daddy who whipped up this deliciously simple recipe when his pregnant wife had morning sickness. And he was kind enough to share it with me. A little sweet from the chestnuts and luscious from the cream, it was light and gentle enough to sooth the tummy. But I like it so much I regularly serve it as a first course during dinner parties. By the way, frozen chestnuts are easy to find during winter, carried year-round by some stores, and always available on the Internet (although the shipping costs are steep). This soup keeps in the fridge for up to four days and much longer if stored in the freezer.

Serves 8

    2 tablespoons (1 ounce/25 g) butter
    1 onion, sliced
    1/2 leek, white part only
    1 green apple, peeled, diced, and cored
    1/2 pound (225 g) frozen chestnuts
    1 celery stalk
    3 sprigs thyme
    1 bay leaf
    1/2 quart (1/2 liter) heavy cream
    1/2 pound (225 g) small celery root, peeled, washed, and cubed
    11 cups chicken broth or water

1. Melt the butter in a big pot, then add the onion and leek and cook at medium heat for about 5 minutes without coloration. Add the apple, chestnuts, celery, thyme, and bay leaf and cook for 10 minutes without coloration. Add the cream, celery root, and chicken broth, bring to a boil and let simmer for about 45 minutes. Remove the thyme and the bay leaf.

2. Blend soup in a blender until smooth.

Sopa de Tortilla (aka Tortilla Soup)

I met lifestyle author and television personality Katie Brown while doing a festive Thanksgiving table demo on her TV show, "All Year Round With Katie Brown" and instantly adored her for her relaxed, empowering, and down-to-earth attitude toward entertaining—and life. A short three years later while interviewing her for a magazine article we got to chatting about how we'd quickly gone from single working girls to married working moms. When I asked her if she'd ante up a recipe for this book she offered this light, spicy, soul-satisfying soup and the following explanation: "This soup is one of my favorites because it brings back fond memories of my kind friend Kerstin, who cooked for me when I was on bed rest while expecting my first child. During this time, the only food I absolutely couldn't stand was spare ribs. I couldn't handle the sight of a spare rib anywhere remotely close to me. But, of course my husband loves them and must eat them at least once a week. It was horrible! I managed to find cups full of comfort in a specific food: tortilla soup. My friend Kerstin would come over and cook for me when I was having awful dizzy spells and stuck in bed. Just the act of her cooking was truly mesmerizing, like a master artist at work, not only therapeutic to watch, but also a joy to know I was being taken care of. She would make this amazing tortilla soup, the only thing that would make me happy on those dizzy days of pregnancy. It's still one of my favorite dishes. Simple to make and tasty, you can dress it with diced avocado, thinly sliced green onions, sour cream, grated cheese, chopped cilantro, and lime wedges. Just make sure not to throw in any spare ribs!" By the way, if you're not into spicy stuff, skip the pepper and you're good to go!

Serves 4 to 6

1 15-ounce (425 g) can whole tomatoes
1 onion, chopped
4 cloves garlic, minced
1 fresh or canned chipotle pepper, seeded
1 48-ounce (1.375 kg) can chicken broth
salt and pepper
6 corn tortillas, cut into 4 inch by 1/2-inch (10 x 1-1/4 cm) strips
olive oil for frying
juice of 1 lime

1. In a blender or food processor, puree the tomatoes, onion, garlic, and chipotle pepper.
2. In a large pot, combine the tomato mixture with the chicken broth. Bring to a boil and then simmer over low heat for 15 minutes. Season with salt and pepper to taste.
3. Fill a frying pan a quarter of the way up with oil. Heat the oil and fry the tortilla strips until they are crispy and golden. Remove them from the oil and sprinkle with salt.
4. Remove the soup from the heat and add the lime juice.
5. Serve garnished with fried tortilla strips.

No Muss, No Crust Low-Fat Quiche

I had the privilege of working with chef and culinary teacher Dana Slatkin on her book, *Summertime Anytime: Recipes From Shutters On The Beach*. Part of the family behind L.A.'s beloved luxury hotel Shutters On The Beach, she is one of the most thoughtful and genuinely sweet individuals I know. She is also the embodiment of my kind of joie de vivre—one that blends the simple pleasures of life and healthfulness with a true sense of celebration, lightheartedness, and decadence. This impossibly fluffy and delicious cheese-soufflé-like quiche is case in point. She told me that during all three of her pregnancies, she got wicked cravings for cheese, especially during the second trimester when calcium was in high demand. This sensationally cheesy—but not too rich or greasy—quiche was her answer. A bonus for the busy mom-to-be is that you can sub any veggies you have handy, so long as they're not watery.

Serves 8

2 tablespoons extra-virgin olive oil
1 large leek, white and green parts, chopped
1/2 pound mushrooms, sliced
1/2 cup nonfat or lowfat yogurt
4 eggs
1 egg white
1 1/2 cups nonfat or lowfat cottage cheese
1/4 cup all-purpose white flour
1/4 cup grated Parmesan cheese
1/4 teaspoon salt
1/4 teaspoon black pepper
1 1/2 cups grated smoked Gouda, smoked cheddar, Gruyere, or Swiss cheese
1/4 cup chopped chives
4 slices smoked veggie Canadian bacon, diced (optional)

1. Preheat oven to 350°F (180°F). Lightly oil a 10-inch (25 cm) pie plate or quiche dish.

2. In a large skillet, heat 1 tablespoon of the oil over medium-high heat. Add leeks and cook until soft, seasoning with salt and pepper. Transfer to a large mixing bowl to cool.

3. Add the remaining tablespoon of oil to the skillet and heat over high heat. Sauté the mushrooms until they are well browned; season to taste with salt and pepper. Add to mixing bowl.

4. Drape a paper towel over a small bowl and place the yogurt on top of it to drain; scrape the yogurt into a food processor or blender, add the eggs, egg white, cottage cheese, flour, Parmesan cheese, salt and pepper, and blend until smooth. Add to mushroom-leek mixture. Using a spatula, fold in cheese, chives, and veggie bacon. Pour into the prepared baking dish. Bake for 40-50 minutes, or until knife inserted in center comes out clean.

Warm Portabello Mushroom and Asparagus Salad

When chef/husband/daddy Josiah Citrin of Mélisse Restaurant in Santa Monica, California, heard I was looking for fun pregnancy craving recipes he anted up this light and lovely salad which he made for his wife and mother of two, Diane. She told me she was particularly fond of the mushrooms because they leant a meaty heartiness to the dish without making it heavy. She regularly munched on it in the backyard during early summer. Perhaps you might enjoy following her lead.

Serves 4

8 white mushrooms
4 cloves garlic
salt and pepper
4 portabella mushrooms, stems removed
8 large asparagus stalks, peeled and cooked
1 diced shallot
1 tablespoon parsley, chopped
3 tablespoons olive oil
1 tablespoon lemon juice
2 bunches baby Italian frisee, chopped

1. Prepare the mushrooms: Preheat oven to 400°F (200°C). In a medium oven-safe saucepan with a lid, place the white mushrooms, garlic, 1-1/2 cups water, and a sprinkle of salt and pepper and cover with portabellas. Bring to a boil, then cover with a lid and braise in the oven until tender, about 45 minutes. Remove the portabellas from the braising liquid, then strain liquid into another pan and simmer until it is reduced by one-half.

2. Prepare the asparagus: Peel asparagus up to 2 inches (5 cm) from the top. Cook in boiling salted water for 7 to 8 minutes or until tender. Immediately transfer the asparagus to an ice-water bath, trim ends, and reserve.

3. Serve: Cut the portabellas into six wedges. Bring the mushroom jus (reduced mushroom water) to a boil, add asparagus and portabellas and heat slowly. When warm, add the shallot, parsley, olive oil, and lemon juice. Season to taste and mix well. Remove from heat. Toss with Italian frisee in a bowl and serve immediately with crusty garlic bread.

Calamares en su Tinta (Squid in Its Own Ink)

I met the incredible Spanish chef José Ramón Andrés, who has multiple restaurants in D.C., during an over-the-top private dinner we shared in the kitchen of Carmel Valley, California's Bernardus Lodge. During six hours of gluttony, I became captivated by his playful attitude, passion for his family, and his take on creative and exciting food, which during future encounters included a genius foie gras-cotton candy combo.

He was kind enough to bestow this Spanish recipe upon me with the explanation that his wife Patricia had strong cravings for it while pregnant with their eldest daughter, Carlota, and demanded it nearly every day. A smart chef, José added it to the menu—with a scoop of white rice, the way Patricia likes it—at his restaurant Jaleo so she could stop by and indulge anytime. Not surprisingly, it's now one of Carlota's favorites, too.

By the way, if squid is not your thing you can easily sub shrimp; according to the American Pregnancy Association, in the realm of seafood, both contain the lowest amounts of mercury.

Serves 4

1 pound (450 g) squid, cleaned
3 tablespoons extra-virgin olive oil
2 Spanish onions, thinly sliced (about 2 cups)
1 garlic clove, peeled
1 bay leaf
1/4 green bell pepper, cleaned and sliced into small strips
1/4 cup white wine
1/4 cup canned tomatoes, pureed and strained
1 cup fish stock or water
1 tablespoon squid ink (available through seafood purveyors)
Salt

1. Prep the squid: If the squid bodies are 2 to 3 inches (5 to 7 cm) in length, leave them whole. If they are larger, cut them in 1-inch (2-1/2 cm) rings. If you prefer, you can cut them into triangles instead, by cutting the side of the body lengthwise, laying the squid out flat, and slicing diagonally across to make a series of triangle shapes.

2. Pour the olive oil into a small casserole and bring to a medium heat. Add the onions, garlic, bay leaf, and bell pepper and cook for 60 minutes, stirring occasionally, until the onion caramelizes. You'll know the onion is caramelized when it becomes soft and tender, with a light brown color. If the onion begins to get dark or starts frying, add 1½ teaspoons of water. This will help cook the onion evenly without burning.

3. Add the wine and reduce by half, about 1 minute. Pour in the tomatoes and cook for another 5 minutes, until the tomato reduces and becomes a nice, deep red color. Pour in the fish stock and bring to a simmer. Add the squid ink, stir together, and remove from the heat.

4. Take out the bay leaf and discard. Using a hand blender, puree the sauce until everything is smooth and thoroughly mixed together.

5. Return the casserole to a medium heat. Season the squid with salt and add to the casserole. Cook for 15 to 20 minutes, until the squid is soft. Serve immediately.

Chicken, Mango, and Avocado Salad
with Spiced Candied Pecans

When I was eight months along, I waddled into a San Francisco restaurant and had a mediocre version of this salad. Enamored of the concept, I went home and created my own recipe, which rocked my pregnant world and stayed hugely popular with visiting friends long after I lost my maternity pants. Elegant, fresh, and guiltlessly indulgent, it's a fast and fabulous one-dish meal that is so freaking good it may just become a lifelong favorite.

Serves 6

2 boneless, skinless chicken breasts
5 tablespoons extra-virgin olive oil
1 tablespoon unsalted butter
1 cup pecans
2 teaspoons plus 1 tablespoon sugar
1/8 teaspoon cayenne pepper
1 tablespoon white wine vinegar
1/2 teaspoon Dijon mustard
1/4 teaspoon salt
8 cups (8 ounces/225 g) mixed baby greens
1 ripe but firm Hass avocado, peeled and cut into cubes
1 ripe but firm mango, peeled and cut into cubes

1. Preheat the oven to 350°F (180°C). Place the chicken breasts in a baking dish, baste them with 2 tablespoons of olive oil, sprinkle with salt, and bake for 30 minutes or until thoroughly cooked.
2. In a medium skillet, melt the butter. Add the pecans and cook over medium-low heat, stirring frequently, until the nuts turn a deep brown, around 5 minutes. Sprinkle the nuts with the 2 teaspoons of sugar and the cayenne and stir just until the sugar dissolves. Quickly transfer the nuts to a plate or piece of tinfoil to cool.
3. In a small bowl, whisk together the remaining olive oil, vinegar, mustard, salt, and the remaining 1 tablespoon of sugar.
4. In a large salad bowl, toss the salad greens with the dressing, season with salt, toss in the avocado, mango, candied pecans, and chicken and serve immediately.

Shrikhand with Yogurt Cheese, Saffron, and Pistachios

Ruta Kahate is a fabulous Indian cooking instructor, author, tour guide, and mom of two. When she forwarded this recipe, which I've adapted from her book *5 Spices, 50 Dishes: Simple Indian Recipes using Five Common Spices* (Chronicle, May 2007), she confessed the following: "I did notice a distinct sweet tooth in my third trimester during my first pregnancy. Thankfully I didn't suffer from gestational diabetes, but I still didn't want to overindulge, especially because it was the third trimester and I could just see all the calories collecting around my hips!" Her solution was this Indian dessert made from yogurt cheese. Had I had it, maybe I could have exercised more self-control, too. Sweetened with sugar and made rich with the addition of saffron and nuts it is virtually guilt free, fulfills calcium needs, and is as creamy and decadent as rich, thick pudding. Note: I'm lazy, so when I first read the recipe I wasn't sure the benefit of draining yogurt overnight. But I tried it and I'll tell you what: If you want an obscenely easy, health-minded, and tasty indulgence, this is it, especially if you use low-fat yogurt (and less sugar since it yields less yogurt cheese). Don't dismay if you don't have all the equipment. You'll need to buy cheesecloth (available at most gourmet stores), but I crushed the cardamom seed with a thick juice glass instead of a mortar and pestal. You can also sub the cardamom and pistachio for whatever rocks your world, which makes this an all-around handy dessert. Try it and thank me later.

Serves 4

2 quarts (2 liters) whole-milk yogurt
3 whole green cardamom pods
1/2 teaspoon saffron threads
1/2 cup sugar
2 tablespoons coarsely chopped raw pistachios

1. Line a large strainer with a double thickness of cheesecloth and place the yogurt in it. Bring the ends of the cloth together and tie into a bundle. Set the strainer over a deep bowl and place in the refrigerator for 8 hours. All the whey will drip away, leaving behind thick yogurt cheese. (Check occasionally to make sure the bottom of the strainer is not sitting in a pool of drained whey. If it is, empty the bowl and reset the strainer on top.)

2. Using the side of a knife, smash the cardamom pods so that the peels loosen. With your fingers, pry out the seeds and use a mortar and pestle or a very clean spice grinder to grind them to a fine powder.

3. Heat the saffron threads in a small skillet over low heat until crisp, but be careful not to burn them. This should take less than 1 minute.

4. Place the yogurt cheese in a food processor. Add the sugar and pulse in the food processor only until the sugar dissolves, 30 to 40 seconds. (Do not overmix or the yogurt cheese will thin out too much. You do not want to whip the yogurt; shrikhand should be thick and creamy in consistency.)

5. Crumble the toasted saffron over the shrikhand, fold in the pistachios and cardamom, and set aside, covered, for at least 2 hours for the flavors to blend. Serve cold or at room temperature. Shrikhand will last, tightly covered in a glass dish, in the refrigerator for 1 week.

Avocado Cream Pie

Cat Cora is one fierce woman. The executive chef for *Bon Appétit* magazine, president/founder of Chefs for Humanity, Iron Chef winner, and TV personality is also a mom of two! Leave it to her to offer me a dessert that actually sounds like a pregnancy craving, takes minutes to make, and tastes so delicious that before I could overindulge, my husband finished half of a pie in one sitting. Cat says, "It's craveable because it is rich, creamy, and yummy, but has a lot of good nutrients, too, because of the fresh avocado." I second those kudos—and love its beautiful pale green look, too. But be warned: this definitely does not fit into any low-fat pregnancy diet. FYI: To toast shredded baking coconut, just put it in a pan over medium heat, stir occasionally, and remove it from the heat the minute it turns golden brown.

Serves 6 to 8

3/4 stick (6 tablespoons) butter
1 tablespoon honey
1 1/2 cups graham cracker crumbs
1 can (14 ounces/400 g) sweetened condensed milk
8 ounces (225 g) cream cheese
2 ripe avocados, peeled and pit removed
1/4 cup lime juice
1 teaspoon vanilla
1/8 teaspoon sea salt
1/2 cup coconut, toasted, for garnish

1. Preheat the oven to 325°F (160°C). To make the crust, melt the butter in a small saucepan, over low heat. Stir in the honey. Add the graham cracker crumbs and mix well. Pat the crumbs evenly onto the bottom and up the sides of a 9-inch (22-1/2 cm) pie plate. Bake the pie shell for 12 to 15 minutes. Remove from the oven and cool.

2. In a medium bowl, combine the condensed milk and cream cheese. Blend well with an electric mixer.

3. Mash the avocados with the lime juice and add to the milk mixture. Add the vanilla and salt, and beat until smooth. Turn into the cooled crust. Garnish with the coconut, cover, and chill for 2 to 6 hours before serving.

Sweet & Salty Cravings Brownies

You will hate me for giving you this recipe, so forgive me in advance. These brownies are so insanely good that it is impossible not to overindulge in them. Considering the source, it's no surprise. The mommy who handed over the secret recipe is none other than Trish Karter, owner of the very outstanding Dancing Deer Baking Company. (If you aren't familiar with their baked bits of heaven, visit www.dancingdeer.com and get ready to drool.) She says, "For ultimate satisfaction, you can stir in 1 to 1½ cups of your favorite add-in cravings. Some yummy ones are bittersweet or white chocolate chips (or both), bits of dried apricots, cherries, and cranberries, and chopped toasted nuts, especially walnuts, almonds, and cashews."

Makes 20 brownies

1 1/2 cups Dutch cocoa powder
3/4 cup all-purpose flour
1 teaspoon kosher salt
3/4 teaspoon baking powder
4 large eggs
2 cups sugar
2 sticks (16 ounces/450 g) butter
1 teaspoon pure vanilla extract
1 8-ounce (225 g) jar caramel sauce or dulce de leche (a caramel-like dessert sauce
 available at specialty supermarkets and Latin food stores; optional)
Sea salt to taste

1. Start with all of the ingredients at room temperature, preheat oven to 350°F (180°C), and grease a 9-inch (23 cm) square baking pan.
2. In a bowl, stir together cocoa powder, flour, salt, and baking powder. Set aside.
3. In the bowl of an electric mixer fitted with the paddle beater, beat the eggs and sugar on high speed until very thick and more than double in volume, about 5 to 7 minutes.
4. Reduce mixer speed to low, add the dry ingredients, butter, and vanilla. Beat until just blended. Pour the batter into the prepared pan and spread evenly.
5. Bake until the brownies are set and a toothpick inserted into the center comes out with a few moist crumbs attached, about 25 minutes. Transfer the pan to a wire rack and let cool completely, about 1 hour.
6. Cut into 20 pieces. For over-the-top yumminess, spoon or pour a generous serving of caramel sauce or dulce de leche over each brownie, and garnish each with a pinch of sea salt.

Chocolate Ice Cream Soda

When I put my all-points-bulletin out about pregnancy craving recipes, I forwarded it to my friend David Leite of the online food mecca Leite's Culinaria (www.leitesculinaria.com). He passed it to Cindi Kruth, his senior recipe tester, who also teaches baking and pastry arts at the University of New Haven in West Haven, Connecticut. She was kind enough to send me this fizzy taste of chocolate heaven along with the following explanation: "When I was pregnant with my son, all I wanted to eat was tomato juice and hard-cooked eggs. I gained a measly 13 pounds. My friends were all worried, but he was fine. A few years later with my girls, however, I craved, craved, craved ice cream sodas—the chocolatier the better. Unfortunately, the concocting of this yummy drink seemed to be a lost art. Nearly every ice cream shop I visited thought I meant a Coke float. The real deal is ever so much more satisfying. And when else in your life can you convince yourself that a giant ice cream drink is ok as an everyday beverage? Hey, it's very nourishing; it's half milk. Twins need a lot of calcium to develop properly. See how easy that was. Oh yeah, I gained over 40 pounds this time."

Serves 1

3 tablespoons chocolate syrup
3/4 cup very cold whole milk (lowfat, if you insist)
2/3 cup chocolate ice cream (3 small scoops)
3/4 cup ice cold seltzer water

1. In a 20-ounce (600 ml) glass, mix the chocolate syrup and milk.

2. Add the chocolate ice cream. Stir well until the ice cream softens and starts to melt into the milk.

3. Add the seltzer. Stir just a little to mix.

4. Top with another scoop of ice cream.

5. Drink up!

The Mommy Menagerie On ...The Pregnancy Diet

I asked 111 mommies whether they followed a special diet that took into consideration the recommended guidelines for pregnancy eating, ate whatever the heck they wanted (including as much as they wanted, whenever they wanted it), or something in between. Get a taste of their responses with the following highlights:

"I felt like my body definitely let me know what I needed. I had never had that feeling before."

"I paid attention to some guidelines, but was more relaxed about others. I ate sushi (as long as the fish had been previously frozen), drank the occasional glass of wine, and ate liver pâté."

"When I was at work, all bets were off. I ate when and what I could. I definitely ate a lot of cookies at staff meals. When I wasn't at work, I ate very well. I love the leafy green veggies. I tried to drink milk, but I only like chocolate milk and even that isn't always appealing."

"I totally ate what I wanted. I added more milk, which works well since it goes with chocolate. I figured that would be good for the baby."

"I think with the first pregnancy I went a bit crazy and drank and ate everything, including chocolate. I gained a lot of weight (which took forever to lose) and with the next one I was a bit better about my intake. No more decaf mochas at Starbucks!"

"I ate whatever I wanted to. Prior to the pregnancy, I didn't eat meat (poultry, pork, or beef), but I did eat seafood. About three months into it, the baby was demanding chicken sandwiches, so I gave in."

"I have a relatively healthy diet, but for exactly two weeks I craved the nastiest cheese puffs--something I would not normally touch."

"In my first trimester I ate really healthy and got my six or seven servings of fruit and veggies a day and didn't eat refined carbs, and STILL gained 11 pounds in 12 weeks. So after that, I gave up and did the 'somewhere in between' diet. If I wanted McDonald's, I ate McDonald's. If I wanted a salad, I ate a salad."

"I ate peanut butter almost daily before pregnancy. After pregnancy I only ate it once a week. I have two pregnant friends who ate a ton of peanuts during pregnancy and then had children who were allergic to peanuts. I don't know what kind of scientific evidence there is on this, but the anecdotal evidence suggested to me that there was a strong tie."

"With my first pregnancy I was very fastidious—I wrote down what I ate to make sure I was getting enough servings of fruits and vegetables, and I kept track of how much protein I ate to make sure I was getting at least 80 grams, but I never restricted calories and ate as much as I wanted. With my second pregnancy I've been much more relaxed. I haven't really kept track but just tried to be generally good about getting a fair amount of healthy food in me, and then I add the cookies or ice cream on top."

"Ate as much as I could of anything. I was ravenous and ate constantly up until seven months; then it slowed down as he was getting on my stomach the rest of the pregnancy and I constantly felt full."

Early in my pregnancy I awoke at the strike of 3am each night for several weeks, for an hour at a stretch. Soon afterward came frequent late-night tinkle trips that had me blindly stumbling to the bathroom where my husband was usually thoughtful enough to have cleared a path and left the seat down. Next followed the sore breasts syndrome, which forced me to throw on a sports bra for bedtime and still gasp and recoil in pain with every toss, turn, or unintentional brush against my husband's arm.

Having plenty of moonlight hours to ponder these new occurances, I decided that my body was performing a baby-nursing fire drill—slowly weaning me from undisturbed sleep so that on that fateful day that our human hunger-alarm began to regularly sound, I'd be prepared to jump out of bed with dual milk hoses blazing.

Briefly, somewhere in the first trimester, sleep was much easier to come by, but so were occasions when I woke from a full night's slumber more exhausted than when I went to bed. On some days moving from the bedroom to the front door seemed too much to endure. I not only completely empathized with children who cry when they are overtired, I joined them with the vehemence of a preschooler whose toy had been yanked from his grasp. The overwhelming sense of exhaustion rendered a can-do overachiever like me into a helpless and panicked puddle of tears.

Thankfully that stint was short-lived but, from the middle of the second trimester on, I never made it through a single video rental, regularly became one with the couch, and, according to my husband, developed snoring skills that could rival an industrial-strength chainsaw. (They did go away after Viva was born.)

Late in the game, bedtime comfort became more of a challenge, although I still passed out like a novice party girl on prom night. A perpetually beached whale, I felt as though I would crush under my own body weight, especially when back pain halted me from readjusting my weight distribution and caused the part of my body that I was laying on to go numb. Waking my husband to roll me over or hoist me for bathroom runs became status quo. Ingesting anything before bed—water included—incited bouts of indigestion and regurgitation, which were placated by propping up my upper half on a pillow to encourage what went down to stay down. On occasion an agonizing leg cramp would strike with the gentle grace of a sledgehammer.

Fortunately, I found a bevy of ways to ensure bedtime didn't become a complete nightmare, and I'm happy to share them here. You should make the effort, too, since sleep is critical to a happy pregnancy and much harder to come by the minute the mountain in your midsection becomes its own entity.

> *"Make your bedroom your sleep sanctuary."*

BEAUTY SLEEP

I don't have to tell you how important sleep is during pregnancy. If you haven't already, you're likely to soon experience bouts of exhaustion that make zombies seem as energetic as NFL cheerleaders compared to you. The way to remedy it? Sleep! And sleep a lot—whenever you need it and have the luxury. While you aren't likely to feel tired for the entire prenatal duration, you will face a variety of changes that require you to continually alter your rest routines. But you can and will look and feel your best—even when you're ready to fall face-first into your soup during dinner—if you create and make the best use of an environment and routine conducive to beauty sleep. Read on for A-list ideas on how to get the best Zs. While some of these tricks will be more relevant early on and others will become important later in the game, all of them can help turn your bed into your best friend.

Rethink your bedroom.

If your slumber spot has also been your romp room and media center now's the time to transform it into the kind of peaceful place where the Dali Lama would feel particularly Zen. In other words, make it your sleep sanctuary where the exclusive activity—other than the horizontal cha cha, if you and your partner are still partaking—is snoozing. If there's a TV in your room, move it to the living room or unplug it. Also scoot your favorite reading chair to another location and clear a path from the bedroom to the bathroom so you won't trip over the mounting pile of dirty laundry during midnight toilet runs. Turn your alarm clock away from you so you can't watch father time creep by in the wee hours. Leave the bedroom window open a crack or more; fresh air will do you good.

Preventing Cramps

No one knows exactly why pregnant women get leg cramps, which can happen in the day but are most noticeable at night. A friend told me if I stayed hydrated I wouldn't get them. While there's no proof that hydration helps, it worked for me; I only got cramps when I didn't drink a lot of water during the day.

Create a good bedtime routine.

My husband and I obsessively watched almost nothing but crime-scene investigation TV dramas during my third trimester. But that was after my bout with insomnia. By this time I was so tired that I would have been able to effortlessly drift into dreamland while a 20-piece orchestra hovered over me and played "Take Me Out to the Ballgame" directly into my ears. If you're more sensitive, you should seriously consider dropping TV dramas, the evening news, and other emotional downers—especially now that you'll be looking at everything through the protective and sensitive eyes of someone who wants the world to be a kind, safe place for their child. (Good luck with managing that one.) Also rethink embarking on riveting novels and catching up on whole seasons of your favorite TV show on video; they can easily seduce you away from snoozeville and push you further into your already spinning head.

Set up a bedside snack bar.

Pangs of hunger or thirst can have you climbing out of bed and into the refrigerator in the wee hours of the morning. Make it easy on yourself by keeping a giant glass of water and easy-to-eat snacks on your bedside table. You can find a good list of pregnancy munchies on page 54, but if you want snacks that further encourage sleep, get milk. The childhood comfort—warm or cold and with or without honey—can soothe your weary soul partially due to nostalgia and also because it contains the amino acid tryptophan, which raises your brain's sleep-encouraging serotonin levels. A bite of turkey, which also naturally contains tryptophan, can do the same trick.

Eat moderately.

Later in your pregnancy you might want to refrain from swallowing half of the refrigerator contents just before bed. If you finish dinner by 7pm, digestion will start long before it can backfire in bed. If you don't know what I mean yet, you will—somewhere along the way you're likely to experience indigestion that makes you feel as though what you

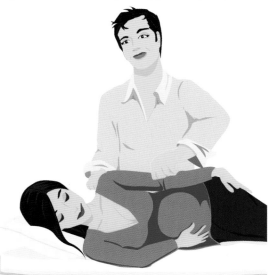

put in your stomach is trying to climb its way up and out. That doesn't mean you should skip a pre-bedtime bite, midnight snack, 1am munch fest, or sunrise nibble. It only means that in the case of the pregnant gal with a gurgling esophagus, less really is more, so eating smaller portions is a big plus.

Exercise.

Your idea of a hard workout may be an afternoon stroll or a two-hour visit to the gym. Even the most modest amount of exercise will do you good, so long as it isn't a 12-ounce curl (repetitive lifting of soda or other canned beverages) or before bedtime. A bit of exercise will help eliminate the day's anxieties and boost your spirits and energy levels during waking hours. For good ways to work it out, see Chapter 8, page 126.

> ### Restless Legs
> Legs feeling fidgety during your last trimester? You're a victim of Restless Leg Syndrome (RLS). It's a common symptom that often happens at night. Experts aren't sure what causes it or what remedies it.

Chill out.

The same things that calmed your crazed and harried soul before you were an ark for one very important passenger are still good bets now, so if you're feeling wound up—or even if you aren't—it's a fine idea to indulge in some pre-PJ pampering. Slip into a nice warm bath. (Remember: not too hot; for specific guidelines see page 26.) Read a trashy magazine or good book. Listen to music or sing, read to, or gently play knock-knock with your bulging tummy, which may just knock back. Or better yet, request a massage from your partner. There's no better time to play the "pamper me, honey" card—so use it while you've got the clout. (That said, it didn't always work for me.)

Get down.

While attending college, I read a newspaper article suggesting that having sex or masturbating was helpful in relieving midterms and finals stress. The same strategy applies to the wide-awake pregnant woman, so if you need an excuse to roll in the hay with yourself or your partner, this is it.

Schedule a Tea Time.

A nice spot of chamomile or Sleepytime tea may help soothe and relax you toward slumber. Whatever you do, make sure you're not sipping tea with caffeine, which is likely to embark you on a quest to rearrange the furniture or decorate the baby's room at 3am.

Dress for sleep success.

Find clothing that increases your comfort. As I mentioned earlier, during my first trimester my breasts hurt so much that in order to sleep I had to minimize their movement by wearing a jogging bra. (This also caused a shockingly robust rash across my chest, which looked much worse than it felt and disappeared quickly with a little airing out.) Later on in the process, I practically lived in pajamas when I was home, slipping into my everyday loungewear and reveling in the notion that I could still fit into my "old clothes." The ruse came to a dramatic end when I sat down and felt a backdoor breeze. I split two pairs of my favorite PJ bottoms before I finally bought comfy, stretchy PJs. If you value your pre-pregnancy bedtime fashions, buy some forgiving PJs or other sleep-friendly clothes in a larger size than you usually wear. You might also benefit from a belly belt or sling, which offers aid to your abdomen and helps your bump back off of your bladder (for details on this undergarment and other wardrobe wisdom, see Chapter 10).

> "Even the most modest amount of exercise will do you good."

Purchase good pillows.

This is not just pillow talk. As your midsection grows there is nothing more soothing for slumber than strategically placed pillows. One between the legs may relieve back pain; one behind your back while sitting in bed—or anywhere for that matter—will also take the pressure off of your spine. One between you and your bedmate can be very helpful if you just want to be left alone. As you grow, your need for pillows will, too, and no fine feathered friend is a better partner for the pregnant woman than the body pillow. Ask mommies about their pregnancy relationship with their five-foot-long fluffy log—or the horseshoe-shaped worm of a pillow called the "Snoogle"—and they're likely to tell you they gave it a name and that it literally came between them and their partners. There is reason for your

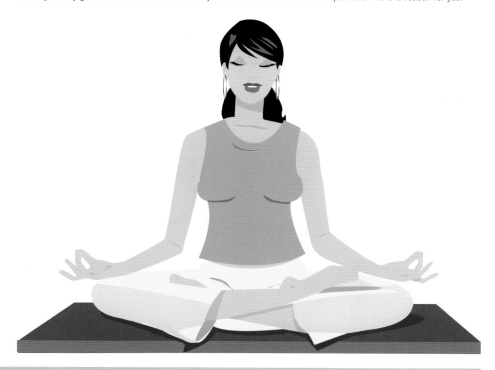

"It's time to calm your mind by thinking of nothing at all."

mate to get jealous. A body pillow becomes your snuggle confident, your comfort, and the one you spoon when you go to bed each night. Should this imposter inspire a pillow fight, reassure your partner that late in the pregnancy you are likely to outgrow it. FYI, you can buy body pillows or Snoogles at most home stores as well as online, see page 183.

Be firm with your bed.

About six months into my pregnancy we got a new mattress, complete with a fancy down pillow-top

Fighting Insomnia

Members of the Mommy Menagerie tell me that for insomnia, some doctors recommended Sominex, which contains Diphenhydramine, commonly known as Benadryl, while others gave Ambien the a-okay. If you're toying with the idea of getting some pharmaceutical aid, don't take anything without consulting a doctor first.

that made our bed look like a sleep-friendly soufflé. I'd tried it out in a hotel when I was just two months pregnant and couldn't wait to make it my central headquarters. Unfortunately, I didn't know that a soft mattress wasn't particularly kind to the pregnant woman until I slipped into its billowing fluffiness only to roll out of bed the next morning with an aching back. Apparently, firm mattresses are better back support for the blimping baby maker. If yours is soft and you want to stiffen it up, slide a wide board under it and ditch the poofy pillow top, if you have one and it is detachable.

Assume the position.

Even before you've truly achieved big mama status, doctors recommend that you don't sleep on your back because when you do your mischievous little fetus and his happy home unintentionally put pressure on your two major blood vessels and impede circulation. Since you surely want your sweet little subletter to breathe easy, you should try to roll your gargantuan self onto your side or spoon your partner or Peter the Pillow. (An argument for the latter: he'll never complain about cold feet or nudge you to get onto your own side of the bed.) Tummy sleepers (myself included) inevitably have to reposition themselves since, after the first trimester, doctors do not advise it and it quickly becomes uncomfortable to lie in bed like a human seesaw. (If you're a side-sleeper they also recommend lying on your left side as much as possible.) Chalk it up as another good reason to turn to gentle and giving Peter who will ease you through the transition.

Just breathe.

If during precious sleep time you're lying in bed thinking about where your child will go to college, what color the baby room should be, or the long list of things you need to do tomorrow, it's time to calm your mind by thinking of nothing at all. How? By focusing on your breathing. Take long, slow, deep breaths, and pay attention to how the air travels through your lungs and to your diaphragm and then exits your body. Follow each breath for as long as you can. If you get distracted, start again, and when all else fails, turn to the next tip.

Do something else.

If you just can't sleep, rather than getting further frustrated, get up and go do something else. Read a book, clean out the refrigerator, make yourself some warm milk, or anything else you like. But keep it relaxing. Watching a brutal boxing match or riveting two-hour movie on late-night TV is not likely to usher you toward dreamland.

The Mommy Menagerie On ...Sleep!

When the mommies were asked about their sleep situations and recommendations, they had plenty to say. Here are some highlights.

"The couch was my friend, although now there's an indentation in one of the cushions! I just kept rolling over on my back in bed which, even though my doctors said it was okay I didn't want to do because of everything I'd read. It also wasn't comfortable. So I had to use the back of the couch for support so I wouldn't roll over. Half of the time I sat up sleeping, which killed my rear end; the other half I was on my left side. I did this for five months."

"I used body pillows, Therm-a-Rest under my sheets, ice packs on my back, and stretching before bed."

"I was so uncomfortable. Nothing helped. You just have to deal. The good thing is you are so tired it doesn't matter."

"Body pillow, U pillow, and, recently and much to my embarrassment AND comfort, Depends. While I can't actually bring myself to pee in them at night, they somehow make getting up to pee that much more bearable. And I haven't found the perfect pregnancy pajamas, but the Depends and a tight T-shirt is great."

"I used Breathe Right strips to help with snoring, though according to hubby, it only helped marginally! No large meals before bedtime."

"When I got bigger my hips got really sore. I got a big foam egg-crate mattress pad. It worked great. I had a lot of trouble with sleeplessness. I found watching TV would put me to sleep, so I made sure I had pillows and a blanket on the couch. I also found that I had to center myself and stop my mind from racing (thinking about all the possibilities for the future) so I could sleep. Meditating helped a lot."

"The very best thing I did for myself was to buy a pregnancy comfort U-shaped pillow. It's body sized and makes you feel like you are cradled in the palm of King Kong's hand. I also liked my back scratcher because for some reason my back was itchy all the time. A good pair of cotton PJs were also good. My best tip is to wear men's briefs (like Fruit of the Loom) when you get really big. They're comfy and provide necessary coverage."

"I liked sleeping alone. For some reason, when I had the whole bed to myself I felt like I could find the positions to get comfortable. I wasn't limited to just one side, I also didn't worry about my tossing and turning that could wake up my husband."

"Early on in the pregnancy when I would go to bed, I listened to Dr. Frank Lawlis's 'Imagery for Relaxation' CD and then, toward the end, his 'Positive Birthing' CD. As a dental hygienist I am more aware of how we can clench our jaws and hold stress in our joints. Even with that knowledge, I needed help to unwind my body at the end of the day."

The Mommy Menagerie's Sleep-Friendly Favorites

I asked my panel for their top tips on how they made sleeping more comfortable as they grew bigger. The results are tried, true, and ranked by the percentage of mommies who mentioned them as best bets for your snoozing pleasure.

31% used lots of pillows propped in various ways.

25% preferred the body pillow.

12% put a pillow between the knees while lying on their side.

8% said they loved the Snoogle pillow.

7% did absolutely nothing.

3% moved to the couch.

2% said it helped to sleep alone.

2% used a U-shaped pillow.

2% relied on their husbands to flip them over.

2% turned to a reclining chair.

2% took Ambien prescribed by a doctor.

2% snuggled their husbands.

2% slept propped up as is done in a hospital bed.

2% found that sleeping while sitting up was the best bet toward the end.

1% took Tylenol PM. (Ask your doctor first!)

1% used a pillow under the belly.

1% bunched her comforter between her legs.

1% used a nesting pillow.

1% made sure to pee before bed.

1% placed a featherbed on top of the mattress.

1% went for a contoured maternity pillow from Bed, Bath, & Beyond.

1% swears by the Tempur-Pedic mattress.

1% loved a memory-foam pad on top of the mattress for extra cushion.

1% added an egg-crate foam mattress atop the usual mattress.

1% added a Therm-a-Rest mattress under her sheets.

1% spent the last days sleeping in a glider rocker.

For me pregnancy was like tropical weather. Most of the time the days were bright and sunny, but every now and then dark clouds would blow in with gale-force winds and cause an emotional downpour so fierce that my husband probably would have nailed boards over our bedroom door if he'd had fair warning. Then, seconds later, the sky would clear and life would become a balmy breeze once again. (At least for me—my husband took a little longer to recover.)

During my first trimester, hunger instantly turned me from my usual perky self to a panicked, mini-mart-ravaging beast. (If only you could have heard the phone call to Colie when I discovered he ate all of my Häagen Dazs chocolate ice cream.) But hormones also worked their voodoo, especially during one morning drive to the gym where for no reason whatsoever I flew into a fit of giggles, fury, and tears all within 60 seconds. It was then that I realized pregnancy was like riding a rollercoaster while blindfolded—I never knew which direction I'd turn and whether my next move would result in screams, laughs, or both.

At just over two months I inexplicably went on a two-week rage. It struck like a lightning bolt and once it hit, I felt that every person, car driver, customer service representative, medical professional, and stranger should either graciously make my life easier or get the hell out of my way. Wherever I went, if anyone within my immediate vicinity did not step aside so that I could pass, I had a severe impulse to throw him or her to the floor. Drivers, unaware of my new rules of engagement, received verbal lashings that would make the most illustrious gangsta rap songs seem clean-cut. Thank goodness my daughter's ears weren't fully developed yet.

I prayed for the day that I would "pop" so that people would know I was pregnant and show me the special treatment I so rightfully deserved—or at least cut me some slack. Of course my rant was over by the time my beer-bellylike pooch evolved to a bona fide baby pouch. Fortunately, I kept most of my pregnancy Tourette's syndrome to myself. But I did not try to squelch it. Instead, I let my boundless ferocity be my muse. It was not only weird to feel impulses of sheer unadulterated rage, it was kind of fun and freeing, especially since I knew it was the hormones talking and not the permanent new me. I had a hall pass to celebrate my inner beast and I took it, deciding that perhaps I was feeling for the first time a mother's animal instinct to

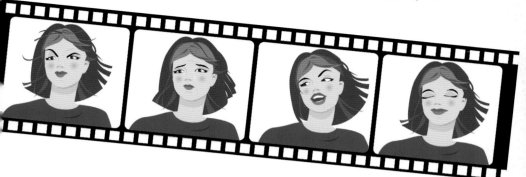

protect herself and her unborn baby—even if it was just from a slowpoke in the gym doorway or an old man blocking the grocery aisle with his cart.

After sailing through the second trimester, I again hit a few emotional squalls on the heels of our birthing classes. Each night after we returned home I cried myself to sleep out of sheer overwhelm, but not before picking a fight with my husband to make the saga that much more of a whole family experience.

Whatever the case, one of the things that got me through the one-woman soap opera of pregnancy was that I embraced all of the mayhem. My perspective was that when my emotions went wilding it was time to enjoy the ride. Rather than judging myself, withholding my feelings, or trying to tame them, I reveled in them, gnashed my teeth, cried my eyes out, and in the back of my mind found amusement and amazement in all of it.

Of course not everyone around me felt similarly entertained or sympathetic when the gestational gloves came off. But I knew that my jabs at the world were not sucker punches. They were legitimate mood swings that diffused some of my hormonal madness with each uncontrolled blow, and I hoped that those around me understood that, too.

If you're feeling uncomfortable with the new wilder you, consider this: Given the amount of work required for your body to build a whole new person from scratch it's not at all surprising that it needs to let off steam. So when that little pregnancy devil takes over your regularly angelic persona, give yourself a break. When you regain composure you can polish your tarnished halo by apologizing to anyone necessary with three perfect-excuse words: "Sorry. I'm pregnant."

LOST THAT LOVING FEELING?

During the course of writing this book several mommies expressed to me how unprepared they were for the emotional side of pregnancy. The physical effects were obvious enough, but apparently not everyone knew that the crazy hormone cocktail the pregnant body is continually swilling can momentarily propel even the most relaxed, jovial mommy-to-be into states of belligerence, hopelessness, or fury over things as trivial as a television commercial or a missing tub of ice cream. Tack on common pregnancy concerns, such as what the future will be like, the state of your fetus's health, strained familial relationships, or how your marriage, job, or friendships will change after you're a mom and you've got every excuse to have full-blown freak-outs on a regular basis.

If you're not feeling funky, don't future trip that you will. Not everyone internally combusts. Some mommies are in a perpetual state of pregnant bliss, others find the experience to be about as fun as an IRS audit, and some cruise through the trimesters hitting the occasional PMS-like road bump with nary a bruise to show for it. But should you find yourself falling into a deep dark hole of sadness, anxiety, fear, or just plain pregnancy insanity, read the following measures that can help you find your emotional footing.

Accept that you are no longer in control

and go with the flow. Recognizing that you are not in the driver's seat and relaxing about it makes for a far easier ride. This general pregnancy truism was best exemplified for me during labor. I was in my hospital room with incredibly intense 60-second contractions that were three minutes apart. As the waves started to hit my first instinct was to jump out of my body and make a run for it. But since that wasn't an option I went with my second choice, which was to brace myself, squeeze my eyes shut, clench every muscle in my body, and resist with every ounce of energy I could muster. However, I quickly discovered that the exact opposite tactic was the best way to get through them. When I felt a contraction coming on I got into the most comfortable position: bent over a tall table with my head resting on crossed arms and my legs spread like a police suspect being frisked. Then I focused on deep breathing and relaxing every muscle in my body, from my jaw to my shoulders to my legs to my toes. Doing a mental inventory and attempting to relax each muscle was a great diversion, made the pain easier to bear, and allowed me the mental capacity to become more fascinated by my body's performance than anguished by it (though that didn't stop me from later requesting an epidural). Similarly, fighting your newfound lunacy is infinitely more exhausting and traumatizing than simply embracing the things you cannot control.

Don't hang out with people who piss you off.

Pregnancy does a funny thing to relationships. It can bring you closer to friends who have children, clarify just how supportive people in your life are, and bring new depth to familial ties. But it can also alienate you from pals who are feeling envious of your new status or don't want you to change, dredge up your childhood grievances against family members, and make usually pleasant enough people seem extremely annoying—especially if they yammer on with unsolicited and unwelcome maternal advice.

In the latter instances my recommendation is to steer clear of irritating people as much as you can. You may not be able to dodge your patronizing boss or grumpy husband, but you can easily put some distance between yourself and that judgmental friend or know-it-all neighbor. Give yourself a little space from stressful relationships and you may even find a place in your heart to be gracious toward them later on.

Spend time with positive people.

It's just as important to surround yourself with people who are upbeat and support your status right now. Seek out sunshine people who can share your excitement with you.

Screen your calls.

Letting the answering machine pick up is an intelligent way to stop yourself from getting worked up by anyone you're not in the mood to talk to. Incidentally, this preemptive measure becomes even easier after the baby arrives when you officially have a lifetime excuse to abruptly hang up without explanation (a huge boon when your mother is nagging you), not answer the phone at all, or take your sweet time to return calls. (Months are not unheard of among friends.) This, ladies, is one of the secret bonuses of motherhood—from here on out you are officially off the hook.

Edit your calendar.

If you've become less Dr. Jekyll and more Mrs. Hyde, an overbooked schedule can make matters worse. Clear your calendar of unnecessary dates during especially emotional stints. That way rather than biting off a seldom-seen relative's head at a business dinner, you can let your inner wild woman loose at home on someone who will still love you tomorrow.

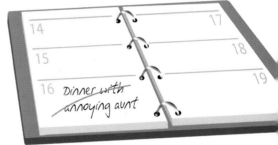

Get some exercise.

Breaking a sweat isn't addictive for nothing. Getting into a workout groove encourages your brain to release endorphins, the body's naturally occurring painkiller that is deployed whenever you are subjected to pain or stress. Try a brisk walk or take a swim. It is likely to put you into a happier headspace. For more exercise information, see Chapter 8.

Watch what you eat.

If you're trying to tame your inner fire-breathing dragon, gulping down sugar, caffeine, chocolate, or all of the above may be like gargling with gasoline. Eliminate foods that can throw your body off balance and see if it helps smolder your emotional flames. For a cornucopia of dining details, see Chapter 3.

Keep food on hand at all times.

One surefire way to incite the wild animal in you is to let yourself get good and hungry. When that happens, pity the fool who stands between you and your next meal. Show mercy on the minions by making sure you have snacks on hand at all times. For a tasty list of portable munchies, see page 54.

Rest!

Everything seems a little harder to bear when you're cranky. Get as much beauty sleep as you can finagle. It'll help you to remain resilient.

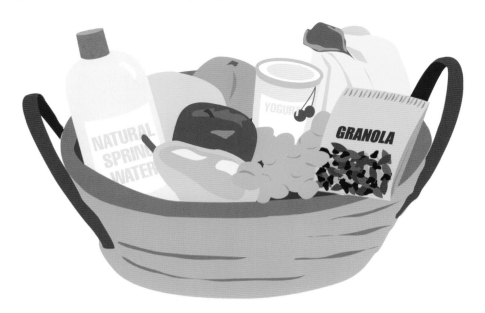

Pamper yourself.

Hormones aside, pregnancy can be stressful—especially since you probably have to trudge through everyday responsibilities regardless of how you're feeling (unless you're on bed rest, which can be stressful for other reasons). Carve out some pamper time just for you—downtime is likely to make you feel better about yourself and give you a refreshed perspective. If you need a pampering primer, you've got it in Chapter 7.

Go ahead and have a good cry.

Long before I became pregnant I fell into a deep depression over some unresolved family issues that were magnified during a trip to Europe with my father. My deadline for my first solo book, *The Last-Minute Party Girl:*

"It's worth cleansing your emotional house whenever the dirt starts to build up."

Fashionable, Fearless, and Foolishly Simple Entertaining was looming and I couldn't type a single word. Struck with writer's block for more than a month, I embarked on walks of my neighborhood each morning, fighting back tears and searching for a lifeline to pull me out of my darkness. When it didn't come, I went to Plan B: I gathered every single pillow I owned, placed them on my bed, and punched and screamed all of my anguish into them until I was too weak to even make a fist. I emerged from the bedroom a new person—lighter, relieved, and borderline giddy as I walked into my office, sat down at my computer, and marveled at how the words immediately began to flow onto the page.

Whether pregnant or not, I believe that repressed emotions can bubble, ferment, and become truly toxic when they're not released. Given that you need all the help you can get right now—and the fact that your fetus feels everything you feel, including anxiety, depression, and anger—it's worth cleansing your emotional house whenever the dirt starts to build up.

While it may not be safe to go full-on Mohammed Ali when you hit an especially rough patch, finding ways to free pent-up emotions—such as screaming into a towel or crying on the bathroom floor, as I did more than once—may be just the ticket.

Watch for deep depression.

It's perfectly okay if you feel like a Jane of the Jungle wildly swinging through the forest of pregnancy emotions while bellowing and beating your newly enlarged chest. But the beauty of mood swings is that they do just that—sway from one end of the emotional spectrum (fear, sadness, anger) to the other (elation, joy, optimism), and usually include plenty of time spent somewhere in between. But if you find that you plunge tummy-first into the deepest parts of your emotional jungle and can't reemerge and see the forest for the trees, seek help from your practitioner. Depression is not uncommon during this very pivotal time (or afterward, for that matter) and a professional is likely to have some ideas on how to pull you out of the pregnancy dumps.

> "Get as much beauty sleep as you can finagle. It'll help you remain strong and resilient."

Don't make any rash decisions

while you're feeling crazed. Making any major commitments while in the midst of hormonal heresy is like getting a tattoo while drunk. Spelling "O-Z-Z-Y" across your fingers may seem like the perfect thing to do while you're riding the crazy train, but the next day you're in for one hell of a hangover—and potentially permanent repercussions. Plainly put, hormones can drastically skew your perspective during the maternity and postpartum months. (I know one mommy who inexplicably couldn't stand her husband for the entire duration, but felt just fine about him afterward.) Make a point of thinking things through and perhaps getting a second opinion from someone you trust before doing anything drastic.

The Mommy Menagerie On ...Maternity Moodiness

I posed the question, "Can you offer a scenario that would exemplify a wild pregnancy mood shift?" Here's what some mommies said:

"I didn't have momentary mood shifts. I think I had long cycles of hormonal swings—a few weeks of sad (boo-hoo), inexplicable rage for two weeks, and then content (resigned?) for the rest of it."

"I was totally psychotic. I was so snappy at my husband it was awful. But the worst part was, I couldn't control it."

"My hysterical laughing. A lot of women cry. I would laugh over the silliest things and not be able to stop. Eventually I would start tearing up, crying, and laughing."

"Honestly, I think I was just cranky through the whole thing. Pretty consistently."

"I didn't have major mood shifts, though every once in a while something super-bitchy would come out of my mouth out of nowhere."

"On occasion, I would go from 'Oh, how wonderful to be pregnant' to 'What the hell am I doing, thinking I can handle this responsibility?'"

"The hunger that would seize me in the first trimester was unreal. I would go from happy mock cocktail girl to snarling starving crazy woman in 60 seconds."

"One minute you are the sweetest person in the world, the next you have realized someone has eaten all the Fruit Loops and left you none and you go hysterical."

"Bursting into uncontrollable tears in a restaurant when I am told it will be a 30 minute wait to get a table."

"Driving on the freeway and having to eat RIGHT THEN and my husband missed the exit to get to the McDonalds. I started screaming at him and then threw a bag of pretzels all over the car because I needed the bag to catch my vomit. Luckily the vomit helped my husband to feel sorry for me instead of hating me for screaming at him."

"Just a general feeling of anger that would come out of nowhere and was generally directed at my husband. It was like watching myself from a distance."

"One minute I would want my husband to be the farthest thing away from me, for no reason at all, I would hate him. The next minute all I wanted was to be like a baby in his arms."

"Screaming at my husband; feeling he didn't care and wasn't giving me and the belly enough attention. Hating him one minute, loving him the next. Ugh."

"I don't remember doing this, but my husband still likes to tease me about it. He calls it 'I love you—what's your problem?!' because that's essentially what I said in the span of 10 seconds. I was all affectionate, like, 'Oh, I'm so glad we're having this baby and isn't it wonderful and you're so great but you do this sometimes (or whatever it was) and I don't understand why you do that—why do you do that? What's your problem?!'"

"My husband sat down and ate an entire jar of pickles one day. I normally wouldn't care, but I got mad and yelled at him for an hour! Over a jar of pickles!!! We still laugh about it to this day."

"My husband would often say when I was moody about something completely juvenile like the weather or something, 'Who took my wife and when is she coming back?'"

"At the end of the day, when I was looking forward to resting, finding out that my husband was coming home late would quickly shift my mood."

"I came home one day from work and I'd had a good day. My mom was supposed to come over to my house that night for dinner and I was looking forward to it, but she was about 30 minutes late. I started to become intensely nervous, obsessively looking out the window, calling her. Then I started calling her friends. I was hysterically crying and convinced she was hurt. Turns out she was just running late at work in the field and her cell phone didn't work where she was."

"My mother and I were leaving to go shopping. I was in a great mood, excited about buying stuff for the baby and she had to run back in the house to get her coffee. I got so mad over having to wait that I had a fit and went home."

"I was about to go into the grocery store with my husband when I ran into a woman with infant twins. Like I always did when I saw a woman with twins, I stopped her to ask how it was going and what it was like. She looked at me wide-eyed as she unloaded her baby girls and said it was really hard. I burst into tears and continued to cry inconsolably throughout the grocery store."

"Sobbing when my husband saw me naked at 36 weeks and he offhandedly remarked how big I had gotten."

"I've been down and very emotional this time around. It's very disturbing to me that I can't seem to get a grip. I feel out of control emotionally and my husband doesn't get it."

"Wild pregnancy mood shifts would usually be precipitated by something really important, like the shirt I wanted to wear being in the laundry, or dropping something I was holding, being out of chocolate, or my husband failing to read my mind."

"I remember needing to re-arrange the house almost on a daily basis in my last two months, and the urgency of it. It was a dire need for some reason. I specifically remember that we were having a nice quiet dinner and I looked into the living room and decided the couch was not in the right spot, so I got up and had to move it and all the other furniture immediately. My husband innocently said, 'Let's just wait until after dinner, hon' and—from my reaction— you would think he had just committed the most horrible sin on earth. I verbally attacked him. I don't have any idea what I said, but I remember his eyes opening wide in fright, and him jumping up from the table to help me, without complaint. We moved that couch about 10 times in the final trimester and it ended up right back where it started. It's the family joke now."

"I didn't know if we should take the perfect apartment because we could not park our car right outside our door. I actually made my husband call our Rabbi and ask him to make the decision if we should take the great apartment or not! He told me to run back and take it and not be crazy."

One of the most harrowing and interesting elements of my pregnancy was the sudden awareness that every little thing I put on or in my body was a big deal. While I'd long been a fan of "natural" beauty products, such as deodorant that does not contain cancer-causing aluminum, I didn't think twice about surrounding myself in a cloud of hairspray on my way out for the night, taking a few gulps of cough medicine if ever I started to hack, or popping ibuprofen at the first sign of a headache. Before reading a smattering of pregnancy books it hadn't occurred to me that some of the everyday things I did could potentially be harmful to my unborn child.

Suddenly it seemed the whole world was a minefield of toxicities that had to be carefully navigated—especially when it came to everyday medications. I winced through a couple of weeks of dull headaches, inspected the occasional acne explosion, and marveled in the unusual aromas wafting up from the nether land. (No need to explain—you'll surely get the drift yourself!) But occasionally I'd forget that my go-to remedies were off limits, like the time my yoo-hoo was so itchy I instinctively slathered it with yeast infection cream, then stumbled upon its pregnancy-warning label and called my doctor in a panic. (No biggie, she assured me. In fact, she later prescribed that very cream for my yeast infections, which plagued me every time I had sex throughout my pregnancy. Fortunately, or unfortunately depending on how you look at it, that didn't happen too often.)

There were also times that precautions were thrown out the window, like at 19 weeks when my back went out for several weeks, during which I literally got stuck on the couch, sobbing in pain and fear until a neighbor came over and pulled me up. I was flat-out terrified when my doctor prescribed Vicodin to ease my pain. With so much alarmist information out there I feared that even one or two doses would compromise the health of my unborn child (an Internet search will quickly unearth a number of credible sources that state no pain medication is 100% safe). Thankfully, it didn't. I turned to Vicodin when the pain really was unbearable but I also found a less-risky remedy more effective: my true savior was a licensed RN/massage therapist who I visited regularly for the rest of my pregnancy.

The point is, if you need medical intervention or took some medication you didn't realize is a no-no, don't stress over it. Just call your practitioner for reassurance and remind yourself that when it comes to pregnancy health, not everything is black and white or always optimal. And in the meantime, try these safe home remedies.

CURES FOR COMMON CALAMITIES

While the Medications Cheat Sheet on page 27 lists a few over-the-counter relief options that doctors give the a-okay, most medicines are no-nos during the baby-waiting game. Still, there's backache, absurdly sensitive breasts, constipation, hemorrhoids, frequent urination, chapped lips, bloody noses, scary skin changes, headaches, gas, mood swings, nausea, vomiting, swelling feet, and stuffy noses to contend with. And those are just a few of the common calamities. So what can you do to mitigate the endless, unfortunate, but totally normal prenatal problems? First, aim for good nutrition as best you can. Anyone who's felt the unpleasant effects of dining on little more than caffeine or sugar for even a day knows how nutrition or lack of it can affect your overall state—and that's without pregnancy hormones kicking in. Second, browse through this chapter for safe, sane, and fast ways to sooth maternity's mental and physical sagas, or at least have a good laugh. And remember that you might need to try more than one remedy or even combine them for results. Third, if you have severe physical discomfort or cannot remedy a problem, contact your healthcare provider for help ASAP.

Now two quick disclaimers: First, this chapter is not meant to freak you out. In fact, if you're the sort who will read about all the possible pregnancy ailments with morbid fascination and then worry about getting them until they either crop up or you give birth, I recommend you skip this chapter and return to it when you actually have a physical side effect and need remedial tips. Second, I'm not a doctor and, while I have compiled insight regularly given by veteran moms and medical professionals (one of whom reviewed these recommendations), any of the advice in this book should not replace a consultation with your healthcare provider. If you are having serious physical or mental issues, or just don't feel right about what's going on with you and your body, seek medical advice immediately. I include this disclaimer not only because we live in a sue-happy nation and protecting oneself from litigation has unfortunately become a necessity in even the most innocent circumstances (like an upbeat pregnancy book), but also because it's a good idea to do everything you can to ensure the health and happiness of you and your fetus throughout your entire pregnancy and beyond. Now then, on with it—tips on how to quell the most common pregnancy ailments—in alphabetical order for easy access.

Acne

If you're having a high-school flashback complete with enough zits to make you want to skip prom, you're not alone. Acne is a common pregnancy problem, which unfortunately cannot—and should not attempt to—be eradicated with mounds of white cream or any other extreme measures. But you can try the following kinder, gentler steps.

Treat your skin with kid gloves. Don't scrub your face with a washcloth or towel. Wash with your hands and pat dry with a towel. Pat your skin dry rather than rubbing it, which can irritate acne.

Wash your face with a mild soap or cleanser twice a day. It'll help cut down on oily buildup.

Exfoliate. Don't go for the medicated stuff without a practitioner's permission. Instead try rubbing oats with water onto your face or dot your damaged areas with all-natural tea tree oil.

Check your cosmetics. Replace moisturizers and makeup that contain oil with nonacnegenic, water-based ones.

Don't pop pimples. It offers short-term satisfaction with potentially long-term scars.

Ask your practitioner for recommendations. If the above suggestions aren't cutting it, don't suffer. Seek additional options, but do not use any medications, over-the-counter or otherwise, without clearing it with a medical pro first.

Anxiety

Feeling anxious about the "what ifs" of pregnancy, childbirth, your relationship, job, or anything else, for that matter? If unsavory possibilities are taking up lots of your headroom, clean your emotional house with the following anxiety-relieving favorites.

Practice meditative breathing. Find a quiet space, breathe deeply into your tummy, and focus on your breathing or a particularly tranquilizing thought.

Exercise. Getting your pulse up is a fantastic form of stress-relief. With its ability to make you feel better about yourself and the world, it's the true meaning of physical therapy. Yoga is an especially good option as it centers your mind and body. Sex isn't a bad option either, if you and your partner are up for it.

Watch your diet. Avoid sugar, load up on protein, which helps maintain even blood-sugar levels, and take a B-vitamin supplement—with your doc's approval.

Seek a sympathetic ear. Call someone you trust with whom you can share your feelings, ideally a person who has gone through pregnancy and might have insight into what you're going through. Or kick it up a notch and join a pregnancy support group or see a therapist or counselor.

Lighten Your Load. You've got plenty on your hands already. Do whatever you can to eliminate unnecessary stresses or responsibilities.

Sleep. Take it from someone who has finally come out on the other side of sleep deprivation—every horrible thought and feeling is amplified when you don't get enough sleep. Give yourself a leg up by getting lots of rest.

Back Pain/Sciatica

During your pregnancy, your pelvis and hips loosen up and your stomach muscles reconfigure in order to make an easier passageway for your downward-headed bundle of joy. Meanwhile, your center of gravity and posture change to compensate for an extra human hanging off of your front side. Given these circumstances, it's no surprise that the back striking back was the number one problem for the Mommy Menagerie. Whether it's aches or sciatica—pains shooting down your lower back, butt, hips, and legs as a result of sciatic nerve irritation—pain may not be altogether avoidable, but it can at least be mitigated. One word of advice: Don't wait for your situation to get dire before doing something about it. Take action at the first hint of an ache. You'll thank me for it later.

Practice prevention. Listen up because this is serious—and a fantastic reason to pamper yourself. The best remedy for back pain is prevention. Great offensive measures include massage, yoga, and osteopathic or chiropractic evaluation, which will let you know how predisposed you are to facing problems. You can also benefit by making sure your weight gain doesn't get out of control.

Stand tall. It's important that you practice good posture now more than ever. Try not to slouch when sitting or standing. Avoid crossing your legs, and if possible, keep them a little elevated. When bending down to lift something, bend at the knees, not the waist, and lift the item close to your body, using your leg muscles rather than your back muscles. Finally, don't sit or stand for too long if you can help it.

Exercise. Keeping your core body strength isn't easy while pregnant, especially if you didn't have much to begin with! But you can help yourself out by safely developing or maintaining a sense of inner stability through your abdominal and back muscles. If you can swing it, hire a knowledgeable trainer to help you. Or try prenatal yoga or light stretching. A nice side bonus: light workouts will help to counterbalance ice-cream weight gain.

Wear a maternity support belt. They're about as glamorous as girdles, but they're also as effective and clandestine, too. Under-the-clothing options include the trochanter belt, which gives circumferential support to the pelvic ring, and a variety of other maternity belts that support the lumbar and abdominal regions by redistributing some of the mother load, so to speak. Ask your doc if a belt is your best bet.

Slip on supportive shoes. Neither flip-flops nor stilettos will do the trick. Shoes with good sturdy support, cushion, and a 1-1/2 inch heel help ease the long road ahead.

Sleep on a firm mattress. Bedtime back support is key. If you don't have a firm sleeping foundation, try sliding a wide board between your box spring and mattress.

Sleep in a winning position. Try new horizontal poses when you hit the sheets; a good bet is on your side with a pillow between your legs.

Apply cold and heat. Alternating ice packs and heating pads or warm baths can be very soothing. If you're worried that heating pads are bad for you, don't be. Conventional wisdom is that they are harmless because they cannot raise your overall blood temperature and current research suggests that their EMFs (electromagnetic fields) don't pose any threat to you or your unborn babe. But if you're paranoid like I was, you can always use a microwavable buckwheat hulls-filled heating pad. (I like lavender, too, but I've seen its strong aroma send a pregnant friend racing to the toilet bowl.)

Reduce stress. There's nothing like a little anxiousness to torque your back. For ideas on how to take a natural chill pill, see "Anxiety" on page 90.

Get massages. Whether your insurance pays for it—sometimes possible so definitely look into it—or you have to dig into your baby's college fund, do not skimp on this restorative experience. When your back is belligerent, regular trips to the massage table can make the difference between a miserable or a magnificent pregnancy. Ask friends or your care provider for referrals to great prenatal-massage specialists.

Try chiropractic work. During one of my pregnancy back battles, a non-force chiropractor strapped me down on a Frankenstein table, lightly tapped my back for a half hour, and sent me on my way. It seemed like a lot of hooey until I realized my back was temporarily pain-free. From that moment on I was a believer. If you seek a chiropractor, get a good referral from your care provider or a mommy friend.

Seek acupuncture. The Chinese practice of attempting to relieve pain or cure illnesses by puncturing specific areas of the skin with tiny needles may ease your aches and soothe your mind.

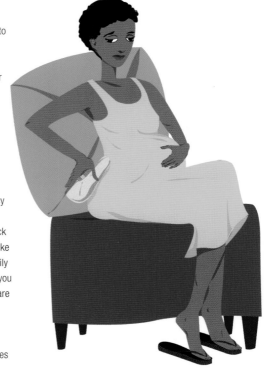

Bleeding Gums

Spitting out red toothpaste that went into your mouth white is more alarming than it is dangerous. Your body's increased blood supply plays prankster in your mouth, causing you to look a little like Dracula after an early morning feeding. What to do? Not much other than the following:

Maintain good dental hygiene. This includes at least one visit to the dentist during your pregnancy.

Be aware. Pay attention to your teeth to make sure you're not mistaking a cavity or other dental problem for a pregnancy peculiarity.

Take vitamins. Take your prenatal vitamin and an extra 500 mg of vitamin C daily.

Have patience. Know that this, too, shall pass.

Body Aches

Your body is going to retaliate—overnight it transformed from a single-serving entity to a two (or more!)-passenger vehicle. But if you find time to partake in the following, you and your achy-breaky body will feel much better.

Take baths. Whether it's hot or cool, a little tub relaxation goes a long way.

Apply heat and cold. Apply a heating pad, hot water bottle, or ice pack to sore areas for 15 minutes at a time.

Reposition yourself. Standing or sitting for too long can wreak havoc on your body. Mix it up a bit—regularly.

Rest. Perchance your body is telling you it's just plain tired. Give it a break whenever you can.

Stretch. Invigorate exhausted muscles by giving them a gentle stretch. See Chapter 8 for exercise information.

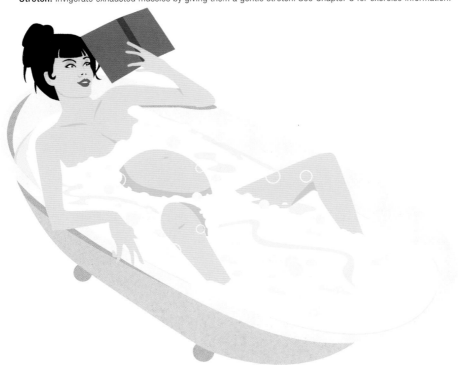

Breasts, Leaky

Unless you're nearing the end of your pregnancy, you're not likely to randomly spring a leak—and even then it's only a possibility, not a sure thing. If you do, it may happen at random or more likely amidst some hanky panky, which is a common titillating trigger so to speak. The culprit of the new juicier you is colostrum, the golden nutrient-rich liquid that your baby will enjoy its first few days of life before your milk comes in. Don't worry, a little spillage isn't going to empty the cup. But you may want to take the following measures to ensure you don't end up broadcasting your bounty on your nice new maternity blouse.

Wear disposable or washable breast pads.

Ease off on the upper-body foreplay—or revel in it.

Breasts, Tender and Swollen

When I was a kid I had "Growing Up Skipper," Barbie's younger sister who instantly grew breasts if you cranked her arm a full 360 degrees. (Can you imagine the uproar that product would garner now?) I felt like her the minute I got pregnant. Overnight I went from a 34B to a 36C—and growing. Only five weeks after conception, I arrived at a holiday party and could tell by the raised eyebrows that there was speculation that I had just splurged on implants. For some pregnant women this baby-induced boob job is a sexy boost to the bust. But if you're reading this section, you probably fall into my camp—forget how it looks, it hurts like hell! Fortunately, the soreness is a short-lived symptom that is likely to disappear during your first trimester. But that doesn't mean you must helplessly suffer through it.

Invest in a new bra. Don't try to cram your new boobs into their old harness. Treat them to the support they need with an honest-to-goodness support bra, ideally one of breathable cotton and good quality that's fitted by a pro. (I bought a cheapie bra on my own, quickly realized that in this instance I'd spare no expense in finding comfort for my bust, and promptly purchased another one from a good lingerie store. It was worth every dollar.) Yes, support bras tend to be about as sexy as grandma underwear, but if your bosom buddies hurt as much as mine did during the first several weeks of pregnancy, you're not likely to feel frisky anyway. If you need to buy a larger size closer to the end of your pregnancy and are planning to nurse, you can save money by investing in a nursing bra, which should ideally be fitted by a pro; it's generally recommended that you buy one size larger than you currently fit.

Handle with care. Soap can dry out and irritate areolas. Skip the suds and rinse them with warm water.

Ice them. When the pain gets bad, apply cold packs or compresses for no more than 15 minutes at a time.

Tell your partner to look but not touch. Recoiling from your partner when he or she tries to touch you is not sexy. Offer fair warning so there's no sense of rejection—and give reminders regularly.

Sleep in a jogging bra or good support bra. Securing your new sensations will eliminate some of the pain that results from repositioning in bed.

Carpal Tunnel Syndrome

Pregnancy-related CTS? Who knew? Some tingling and numbness of the extremities is normal during the gestational journey, but for many mommies-to-be, so is this unwelcome, nerve-compressing side effect that takes hand and wrist pain to a whole new level. Often caused by overuse of the area (think typing on a keyboard) along with simple water-retentive swelling, it manifests itself in numbness, burning, and pain in the hand, wrist, and possibly lower arm.

Irritation may increase at night when your body relaxes and redistributes the day's downward draining water retention. The good news is that this is usually easily relieved—and usually disappears on its own not long after you give birth.

Wear a wrist splint. Available at most drugstores and very affordable, they work wonders.

Help control swelling. See "Swollen Hands, Ankles, and Feet" on page 107.

Ice the area. It may decrease inflammation.

Minimize overuse. If you can't avoid the computer or repetitive motions that irritate the area, take lots of breaks and shake out your hands anytime you feel pain.

Ask your practitioner about supplements. Some natural supplements may help reduce swelling and ease your pain. But don't take anything without medical advice and approval.

Chapped Lips

It seems so trivial until your smacker suddenly gets dry and cracked enough to make a mummy seem moisturized. There's only one thing to do: Arm yourself with lots of lip balms and scatter them in all the places you might need them—by the bed, in your handbag, in the car, and at your desk.

> "Give yourself permission and time to relax when you need it."

Congestion

If you're the proud owner of a schnoz that gets stuffy or develops allergies while you're pregnant, don't sniffle about it and definitely don't take antihistamines, allergy medicines, or use store-bought nose drops or sprays without chatting with your doctor first. Instead try the following; they're not permanent remedies, but they give temporary relief.

Give yourself a facial steam. Get your steam from a hot shower, teakettle (carefully!), or crank up a humidifier. Vaporizers do the trick, too, so long as you keep them clean— they are a breeding ground for mold and bacteria.

Avoid anything you think you might have developed allergies to.

Use salt-water nose drops. To make the drops, dissolve 1/8 teaspoon of salt in 1/2 cup of warm water. Make a fresh batch for each nasal cleansing.

Take Plain Sudafed. While a perfectly pristine pregnancy world is pill-free, the pros at San Francisco's California Pacific Medical Center give this congestion-tamer the thumbs-up. However, no other Sudafed products are approved. Ask your practitioner for more details.

Constipation

One of my least favorite symptoms, constipation is a hard fact of pregnancy (pun intended). It may be caused by the natural and expected slowing of your digestive system or the displacement of digestive organs as your uterus expands. It can also be an unfortunate side effect of taking iron or calcium supplements. It can be exacerbated by what you eat, how you feel emotionally, or how much liquid you drink. There's no easy way around it—over-the-counter laxatives are not an option—but you can take steps to lessen its strain, so to speak.

Feast on fiber. Whole grains (oatmeal, brown rice, and whole wheat bread), raw or cooked fresh fruits and vegetables, and dried fruit may help move things along. Sprinkle some unprocessed bran on your breakfast cereal or nibble on dried fruits. Mmm-mmm!

Drink water. You should be making sure you're hydrated anyway, but perhaps this preoccupation will give you an extra kick in the pants. Drink at least eight eight-ounce glasses each day. A couple of shots of prune juice can help, too. Bottoms up!

Exercise. Yet another reason to get your heart rate going. Take a brisk 30-minute walk or take a yoga class and your bowels may get moving, too.

Ask your care provider. Tell him or her the type of vitamins (if any) you are taking and see if some supplements can help. He or she may also recommend Colace or Metamucil, as San Francisco's California Pacific Medical Center does, or stool softeners or enemas, but do not take anything without a professional opinion.

Edema

See "Swollen Hands, Ankles, and Feet" on page 107.

Exhaustion

Here's the deal: Pregnancy is tiring! You don't even need to get out of bed to feel the strain of your three-trimester, full-body workout. Make it easier on yourself with the following tips.

Relax. Give yourself permission and time to relax when you need to. If you're feeling guilty or badly that you don't have more energy, consider that growing a whole new person from scratch is hard work! On a particularly tiring day you may feel like you haven't done anything, but rest assured: Your innards may have put the final touches on a new set of lungs, just whipped up a perfect set of fingers or toes or grown a liver. And that's no small feat!

Take naps! If you're sleepy, you need sleep. Take a midday snooze when your schedule allows.

Skip caffeine. Contrary to its energy-inducing rep, it can increase fatigue.

Nourish yourself. Do your best to snack on nutritious foods, drink enough water, and take your prenatal vitamins. Low caloric intake and crash-inducing foods such as refined foods, sugary items, and caffeinated beverages may do more harm than good for the sleepy mommy-to-be.

Exercise. It'll boost your energy and good spirits. For details on good ways to work it out see Chapter 8.

Eliminate stress. Whenever possible, give yourself a break. Rather than saying yes to extra jobs, social events, or personal responsibilities, take a rain check whenever possible.

See Chapter 4. It's a whole section dedicated to sensational sleep.

> **About Alternative Medicines**
>
> "Alternative," "herbal," or "natural" medicines aren't automatically safe and healthy for you right now. If you're partaking in any CAM (complementary and alternative medicine), discuss it with your practitioner to ensure it's all good for you and your baby.

Faintness and Dizziness

These common ailments can be due to various body changes, as well as rapid movement (like jumping up from the couch when you suddenly remember you have a secret chocolate stash), and even low blood-sugar levels. If the remedies below don't work, do have a chat with your practitioner.

Eat some protein. It'll stabilize your blood-sugar level.

Easy does it. Get out of bed or off a chair slowly, whether dashing for chocolate or racing to the bathroom.

Get some fresh air. Stuffy rooms or overheating can make anyone feel funky!

Feet Growth

Now's not the time to splurge on a new pair of shoes, unless they're specifically a pregnancy purchase. Over the course of your gestation adventure your feet are likely to swell and spread thanks to loosening joints, and even become a little chubbier along with the rest of you. While many mommies-to-be return to their original shoe sizes, some feet fight the temptation and remain larger for life. (Should this be your foot fate, hook a sister up with your best outgrown boots, shoes, and sandals and you'll have a friend for life.)

Forgetfulness

I consider myself a very responsible person and have been known to give myself grief for losing anything, anywhere, for any reason. Thus, it was quite a shock that at five weeks into my pregnancy, during the mad holiday shopping dash, I lost my credit card—for the first time ever—not once but twice within one week. If forgetfulness is on your symptoms schedule, welcome to the wild world of pregnancy hormones. You may forget the names of good friends, an appointment you made earlier in the day, or where you placed your keys—for the gazillionth time. If that happens, don't sweat it. It's a temporary situation—one that isn't even likely to last all three trimesters.

Write things down. While you may not be able to sidestep random acts of forgetfulness, you do have one defense: Write down everything you want to remember, from questions to ask your practitioner to grocery items to work to-dos. It'll save you lots of stress.

Snack regularly. Keeping your blood-sugar level balanced may help keep your mind centered, too.

Take your prenatal vitamins. Some of the vitamins in your supplement boost mental acuity.

Give verbal confirmation. If you're prone to pointlessly panicking—perhaps about whether you forgot to turn off the stove, let in the cat, or blow out a candle before leaving the house—try a little trick that helped me alleviate paranoia long before I got pregnant. The minute you complete an important task, tell yourself out loud in a big confident voice that it has been done: "The burners are off." "The cat is in." "The candle is out." This simple little exercise changed my life.

Gas

Frankly put, there are no words to adequately describe the potency and shockingly far-reaching residue of a blue-ribbon pregnancy fart. If you've got the kind of relationship with your partner where the occasional game of Dutch Oven is well received, I promise you that during the course of your pregnancy, more than one of your emissions will make you the reigning champion—for life. Alternately, if you are the more modest sort who'd rather sneak out of bed and into the bathroom for private relief, you'd better get over it quickly. If your experience is anything like mine, there will be episodes that make you wonder whether your houseplants or neighbors will survive your latest emission, never mind the person lying next to you.

But there's more to three trimesters of toots than impressive tambour and nose-hair-singing aroma. It's called pain. During pregnancy, your body has higher levels of progesterone, a hormone that relaxes your body's smooth muscle tissues, including your gastrointestinal tract. This relaxation slows your digestive system and can consequently produce enough gas to make you feel as though you're a walking bottle of soda pop—complete with seriously uncomfortable bloating, disabling gas-related cramps, fierce flatulence, excessive burping, and loud gurgles that bubble up into your throat or force their way out the other direction.

You may not be able to completely silence your backside—or very vocal throat or tummy—but you can muffle the madness with the following ideas. Oh, and by the way, this is one instance where the pregnancy stuffy nose really comes in handy.

Identify tummy triggers and avoid them. Learn which foods may aid in tear-inducing gas and limit their intake, especially when you know you're not going to be in the right physical or mental space to air things out. (Trust me, during a company meeting is not the time to discover that filling up on garlicky hummus could inspire your backside to spontaneously trumpet with the gusto of jazz great Louis Armstrong—and be accompanied by aromas that can clear that room faster than a four-alarm fire.) Instigators vary for each person, but notably fart-friendly foods include beans, Brussels sprouts, cabbage, dairy products (for those who have trouble digesting them), garlic, fried foods, onions, and not surprisingly, carbonated drinks.

Practice proper food combining. Had I studied up on food combining during my third trimester I may not have inhaled giant plates of take-out chicken enchiladas with beans, rice, and sour cream and then let my husband's nostrils pay the price. (Then again, who am I kidding?) Regardless, no matter how pretty that array of food looks on the plate, once chewed and swallowed it all ends up in one big pot—your tummy. Some food combinations make for easier digestion than others. And some combinations encourage your food to mingle, ferment, and fight back in the form of seriously gnarly gas. One of your best battles against gas is to eat digestion-compatible foods together and avoid creating tummy clashes. Here are the basic rules of engagement: Eat high-starch foods (pasta, potatoes, rice) with low-starch foods (broccoli, peas, celery, green beans, tomatoes) and eat high-protein foods (meats, beans, seafood, dairy) with low-starch foods. In other words, don't combine high-starch foods with high-protein foods. That means that if there's a rumble in the jungle, a burger, fries, and a milkshake is not your best bet. While we're at it, it's a good idea to avoid combining fruit with high-starch or protein foods, too.

Don't eat big meals. Rather than three big meals, snack on six smaller meals throughout the day.

Eat slowly. Gulping can cause you to swallow air and your tummy doesn't need any more than it already has.

Chew your food. Your parents' sound advice means more now than ever; ingesting slowly and chewing your food well makes food breakdown and digestion easier on your body. It will also help counter constipation.

Don't drink a lot during meals. Adding liquid to the tummy while eating only makes digestion harder. Drink a little bit with meals, but drink more between them.

Eat sitting upright. Sorry. I know it would be ideal to have your partner fan you and feed you grapes as you recline on a chaise, but when gas is bubbling up it's best if you let gravity help what goes down to stay down.

Eat long before bed. Lying down doesn't help with digestion. If you must snack before bed and then feel funky, prop yourself up on pillows so that your head and chest are raised; it encourages food to go with the gravity flow.

Wear comfy clothing. I don't have to tell you how uncomfortable a tight belt feels when your belly is bloated. Do yourself a favor and dress for optimum comfort—especially when you eat.

Exercise. Yet again, exercise comes to the rescue. A brisk walk, yoga, or even meditative breathing can help speed your digestion, calm your head, and limit the opportunity for gas to bubble up.

Turn to the pros. When all else fails, ask your practitioner about over-the-counter gas remedies.

Headaches

Blame it on hormones and increased blood volume—again. Among myriad other things, this dynamic duo can cause dull, persistent, and very pesky headaches. Mine only lasted for a few weeks during the first trimester. Hopefully the same will be true for you. But if you have severe headaches, definitely call your practitioner. If you try to go it alone, forget aspirin and other pain relievers—definite no-nos—without specific consent from your practitioner. Instead, try these combatants:

Prevention. Determine anything that causes or exacerbates them (for example: caffeine, sugar, husband) and avoid those things. Get plenty of rest, eat a number of light snacks throughout the day, and drink lots of water.

Apply hot or cool. Treat your head and back of your neck to a cool or hot compress, depending on your preference.

Relax. Give yourself a time out in a quiet, dimly lit place, or get a massage from a pro or your partner.

Get some air. Stuffy surroundings can make matters worse; change your scenery and breathe in fresh air.

Check with your doctor about regular-strength Tylenol. My practice gave it the a-okay for headache relief, but said all other Tylenol products were definitely off limits.

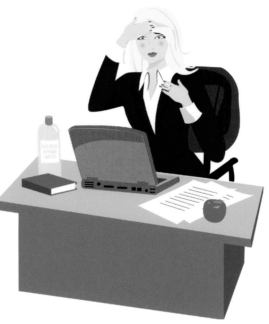

Heartburn and Indigestion

If you burp a lot or feel a burning sensation in your chest shortly after you eat, you can thank hormones or pressure from your tot on your tummy or both. They are the reason your stomach acid and partially digested food can creep up from your stomach into your esophagus and cause severe discomfort. It's normal, for sure, but definitely no fun. Fight back with the following:

See "Gas" on page 97 and follow the recommendations for quelling it.

Mommy Heartburn Tip

"The worst thing I felt physically was heartburn. At times I thought I was having a heart attack, and there was nothing I was able to do, no position I could be in, to relieve it. One night, my husband and I were lying in bed and I just sat up quickly and felt like there were knives coming through my chest. I couldn't breathe well and just felt horrible. He jumped out of bed, said, 'Hold on, I'll be right back!' and ran upstairs to the kitchen. He came back down with a big glass of ginger ale and told me to pound it down. I did, and then let out this enormous belch that seemed to shake the foundation. I immediately felt better and asked him how he knew about that trick. He said he saw it on the television show 'ER.'"

Along with gassy no-nos, avoid the following foods. Chocolate, processed meats, coffee, creamy foods, and acidic foods (think citrus fruits, tomatoes, or tomato sauce).

Coat your tummy. Before eating, sip sparkling or still water, milk, or papaya juice or down a dab of yogurt, ice cream, or cream.

Call your practitioner. Ask for recommendations for specific antacids that are safe to take, low in salt, and don't contain large amounts of potentially harmful minerals. Mine said Gelusil, Mylanta, Pepcid AC, Tums, and Zantac were fine.

After meals chew any gum except mint flavors. Minty treats are rumored to increase heartburn potential.

Don't smoke. You already know smoking isn't good for you or a growing fetus, but perhaps you didn't know it also increases heartburn.

Flap your wings. Not just for the birds, raising and lowering your arms may help your heartburn. Quickly raise your arms, bringing the backs of your hands together overhead, lower them, and repeat. (No need to quack, unless it brings you pleasure.)

Hemorrhoids or Rectal Bleeding

I know. The idea of varicose veins breaking loose in your caboose is absolutely horrifying. But these creepy pregnancy culprits—caused by pressure of the growing uterus, increased blood volume, blood stagnation as a result of slowing your activities, constipation, hormones, and pushing out a baby—are very common and often hereditary. (In other words, if your mom didn't get them, it's likely that you won't either.)

No need to ponder whether you have them. There's no mistaking these unwelcome underside invaders. Whether

Mommies on Hemorrhoids

Of the 98 members of the Mommy Menagerie who talked hemorrhoids, 37% got them during pregnancy, 14% found they appeared after pushing during childbirth, 48% didn't get them at all, and 1% instead reported anal fissures (splits in the lining membrane of the anus, which causes bleeding and pain).

they're internal or poking out of your poo-hoo, they result in itching, burning, and light bleeding. Don't worry, they are not harmful to your fetus, but they can be a severe pain in the ass—literally. While unfortunate recipients may not be able to contain them, they can do their darnedest to make the assault a little more bearable. How? Try the following:

Practice prevention. Ask your mom if she had pregnancy-induced hemorrhoids. If so, a little prevention goes a long way. Heed the guidelines below before your bottom starts betraying you.

Avoid constipation. It makes matters worse. See "Constipation" on page 94 and follow the food-flowing rules.

Change your diet. Eat a high-fiber diet, drink lots of water, and devour dark berries, which have high levels of vitamin C with bioflavinoids—a combo that helps capillaries heal. Also partake in pineapple, which combats fibrin, an unwelcome blood element that settles near your itchy source and blocks your blood from flowing freely.

Balance standing and sitting. Don't do either for too long a period. Take breaks and either get up from your chair and move around or have a seat after standing for any stretch of time.

Don't strain yourself. If you're having an unsuccessful toilet tryst, don't try to force the issue. Relax and breathe your body into cooperation. If it just isn't happening, don't sit it out. Come back later.

Take hot baths. Mommy Menagerie members say this helps ease the discomfort.

Break out ice packs. The cooling sensation may temporarily relieve pain.

Use witch hazel. Witch hazel pads (available at most pharmacies) may combat the itchy pain and reduce swelling. For extra relief, refrigerate them beforehand.

Ask your practitioner for recommendations. Some bulk-producing laxatives, prescriptions, or over-the-counter remedies are recommended. But don't take anything without your trusty practitioner's approval.

Indigestion

See "Heartburn and Indigestion" on page 98.

Insomnia

Sleep sagas can start early on in pregnancy then subside until your third trimester when Large Marge status can again wreak havoc on your rest schedule. For slumber suggestions, see Chapter 4, which is completely dedicated to ways to get your snooze on.

Itchy Skin

If your tummy or boobs itch incessantly or intermittently or you've developed welts during the tail end of your last trimester, blame it on your stretching skin. There's nothing you can do to stop it from drying out and going the way of a blown-up balloon as it expands to accommodate your new size. But with these simple remedies you can ease the desire to scratch as shamelessly as a chimp with mites.

> ### The Linea Nigra or Black Line
>
> If you've got a dark line stretching from your pubic bone to your belly button, say hello to your temporary linea nigra (a fancy term for "black line"). Previously your linea alba, or hardly noticeable white line, it lingers through pregnancy as do newly darkened areolas, freckles, moles, and possibly even sections of your face (a.k.a. the "pregnancy mask").

Grease up. Keep the skin moisturized as best you can. Members of the Mommy Menagerie swear by organic olive oil and Palmer's cocoa butter. I stuck with a homemade pregnancy body balm crafted by a perfumer friend. Lotions will work, too.

Take the occasional colloidal oatmeal bath. Collidal oatmeal is extremely fine ground whole oats, which is known to relieve itches and soothe skin. You can make your own, if you grind the heck out of oats with a coffee grinder (essentially to powder form) and drop a couple of cups worth into a warm bath. But you can just as easily buy Aveeno Oatmeal Bath from pharmacies. For optimum relief, make sure the bath is warm, not hot, and gently pat yourself dry afterward.

Avoid hot showers. Yes, they're great, but they can dry out your skin, which may contribute to overall itchiness.

Contact your caregiver. If you've got severe itching anytime, especially during the final months, give your doc a call.

Leg Cramps

No one can say for sure what causes leg cramps. Some say it may be a calcium imbalance, others argue it's a lack of good circulation, and then there's the theory that pointing your toes while stretching in bed springs a cramp into action. But one thing is certain: If you get one, you will know it. It feels like an instant Charlie horse and fortunately goes away rather quickly. Still, they're unpleasant enough that they're worth avoiding. Try the following practices and see if they work for you. Even if they don't, they're good general pregnancy guidelines.

Drink water. A friend told me that if I stayed hydrated I would not experience leg cramps. There's no medical proof that this is true, but I can say that I only got them twice—in the middle of the night—and both instances happened after days when I knew I should have drank more.

Make sure you're not calcium-deficient. One theory is that a lack of calcium causes cramping to kick in. To get at least 1,000 mg into your daily diet, you can enjoy a few glasses of milk, or munch on green leafy veggies, tofu, or broccoli.

Exercise. It's a great way to jumpstart your circulation.

Elevate your legs. You should be doing this anyway; it helps the blood that's been pooling in your lower legs to get circulating.

Flex, don't point. Now's not the time for any on-point ballet moves; when stretching, avoid pointing your toes. Instead, pull your toes upward and push your heels away from your body to get a nice stretch of the calves.

Start a bedtime routine. Take a warm bath and stretch your calves before crawling under the covers.

Moodiness

What? You aren't loving the new emotional you? If hormones have got you feeling blue or seeing red and you aren't happy about it, see Chapter 5 for tips on how to embrace your inner wild child or perchance mellow her out.

Morning Sickness

You know and I know it's not merely during the morning when this sickness occurs. So let's call a spade a spade! Forget this misnomer and see "Nausea" below for myriad coping measures.

Nausea, a.k.a. Morning Sickness

During my pregnancy I had just a few moments early on where an instantaneous and unsolicited dry-heave made me feel like a cat with a blade of grass stuck in my throat. (The smell of coffee was a good yack-inducer.) But for some women, nausea can occur at any time of day and continue for months, though it often subsides after the first trimester. If you're reading this section you don't care about the when, where, what, and why. All you probably want to know is, "HOW DO I MAKE IT STOP?" Try everything below in various combinations, ask your practitioner for other ideas, and when all else fails, remind yourself that while torturous, this really is temporary.

Eat first thing in the morning. Prep your bedside with an inoffensive snack before you get out of bed and eat it before you even pull back the covers.

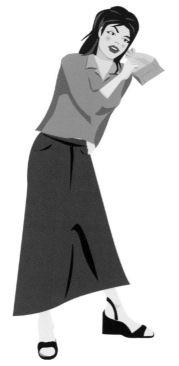

Avoid sudden movements. Whether it's getting out of bed or answering the phone, go slow.

Don't ever wait for hunger to eat. Eating multiple times throughout the day—including just before bedtime—may stop you from continually bending over the nearest wastebasket.

Have food handy at all times. There's nothing worse than attempting to find something to eat when you are seriously on the verge of a hunger-induced breakdown (it's also the number-one way to find yourself crying into the speaker at your nearest fast-food drive-thru). Stick snacks everywhere you might need them—in the car, your purse, desk drawer, bedside, or pocket. Easy-going examples include dry bagels, crackers, rice crackers, nuts, granola bars, and anything else that doesn't make you want to hurl. (For a tasty snack list, see page 54.)

Try these food remedies. All things ginger have been known to quell the queasies, whether it's food prepared with fresh ginger, pickled ginger, ginger drops, or ginger candies. Hard candies, such as Jolly Ranchers, are also mommy favorites, as are foods with high water content, such as watermelon, citrus fruits, and popsicles.

Steady your blood-sugar level. A high-protein diet helps here. Think chicken, fish, cheese, vegetables, beans, and tofu. Other tummy tamers include crackers, breads, rice, potatoes, and even fruit.

Avoid these foods. Fried foods and grease may normally be a girl's best friends, but they aren't easy on the digestive track or the nauseous

The Mommy Menagerie On ...Nausea

What words of wisdom do the mommies have for the sickened pregnant woman? Read on for some of their favorite ways to cope.

"I threw up every time I brushed my teeth in the morning. Leave a toothbrush in the kitchen so you can brush your teeth AFTER you grab a small bite to eat. That always helped me."

"I ate Skittles and Starburst during the morning sickness months, just so what came back up was fruity-tasting."

"Try to eat protein as early in the day as you can stand it. Peanut butter or eggs worked for me. Lemon drops were also very soothing, although they make your teeth fuzzy. Mint toothpaste was a big no-no for me, so I switched to cinnamon."

"If I felt nauseous when I woke up, I kept crackers on my bedside table to get something in my stomach before even getting out of bed."

"Any of the 'Eat crackers in bed before you get up' stuff didn't work for me. The Preggie Pops sometimes did, as did Zofran." (Note: Zofran, or its generic name ondansetron, is a medicine prescribed to prevent nausea and vomiting caused by circumstances such as surgery or cancer treatments. Other alternatives include Phenegan and Compazine. As with all medications, these should be prescribed by your physician.)

"I found if I managed not to move and continued snacking I could stave off the puke. However, it is extremely difficult to do that every minute of every day. It was a tough two months. If you get anything similar, don't try and be tough. Say no to dinner parties and restaurants until you get through the worst. You'll be doing everyone a favor."

pregnant woman. Spicy foods should also sit on the sidelines, as should any and all culprits that make you feel funky.

Drink your dinner. It may be that sipping something is far easier than eating. If that's the case, party on with a thick shake, nice soup, or glass of fresh-pressed veggie juice.

Monitor your liquid intake. Drinking water, other beverages, or soup is great—and especially important if you're losing liquid due to vomiting. It's better to do it between meals, not with them, to aid easy digestion.

Drink these potions. Carbonated sodas, such as bubbly water, ginger ale, and lemon-flavored sodas can perk up your palate, as can pregnancy-safe herbal teas such as ginger, peppermint, or spearmint.

Wear an acupressure seasickness bracelet. These wristbands have been known to help steady the stomach. There are no known side effects and they are available at most drugstores.

Pucker up. Sucking on a lemon or smelling its refreshing scent can temporarily tame the tummy.

Take your prenatal vitamin—if you can stomach it. No doubt swallowing a horse pill is not your idea of a good time right now, but it is worth a shot since you may be barfing up much-needed nutrients. Swallow it at bedtime with a snack, when it's less likely to stage its own curtain call.

Control your environment. Stuffy rooms, heat, and humidity can make matters worse, so try to get fresh air, sleep with the window open, and stay cool.

Chill out. Stress and lack of sleep can only contribute to an unsteady you. Take every opportunity to rest and avoid anxious situations.

Try acupuncture. The Chinese practice of gently puncturing specific points of the skin with needles may not completely eradicate nausea, but it has been known to help and can be quite relaxing if you're not needlephobic.

Ask your care provider for help. If you're losing weight, unable to keep down what you swallow for more than a day, or generally feel miserable, contact your practitioner. He or she may recommend B5 or B6, or a specific medication. Also ask about ginger tablets and wild yam root tablets or extract, herbal remedies that have been known to help.

Nosebleeds

One thing's for sure. During pregnancy, your nose knows. Its sense of smell is so heightened and sensitive that you may be able to describe what your neighbor is making for breakfast from two blocks away. Another common feature is swollen nasal membranes, which are caused by your body's increased hormones and blood volume and may inspire the kind of bloody noses rarely seen outside of the boxing ring. Here's how to help:

Use a humidifier. It'll moisturize your membranes, especially if the air in your home is dry.

Moisturize your nostrils. Apply a light layer of petroleum jelly inside each nostril before bed.

Nausea Stats

Out of 116 Mommy Menagerie pregnancies, 65% came with pregnancy nausea.

Get enough Vitamin C. This supplemental superpower that promotes tissue strength is best ingested through food. Ask your care provider before taking any supplements.

Overheating

There is nothing like heat to suck the vitality out of a pregnant woman. I was due in mid-August—the most popular month for giving birth, by the way—which meant I got to weather the fierce heat of summer while toting 40-plus pregnancy pounds. On the most sweltering days I could only compare myself to a melting ice cream cone. Everything felt drippy, from the sweat droplets running down the backs of my legs to my energy level, which seemed to plummet with each jump of the thermostat. I was fortunate to have access to an unheated swimming pool, and there were a number of days that my husband came home to find me standing in it, chest high, eyes closed and facing the sun. On the days that I was too melted to trudge the 20 steps to the pool, I found solace in huge glasses of ice water, cool showers or baths, and places with air conditioning (movies are a hot-day savior, provided you bring a couple of pillows). If you're feeling like your goose is cooked, I suggest you do the same.

Sciatica

See "Back Pain" on page 90.

Sense of Smell, Intensified

It's official. Your motherly instincts have kicked in and you are now a two-legged bloodhound. What's the pregnancy purpose for being able to sniff out a rank odor, slice of bacon, or cup of coffee from a block away? An evolutionary hand-me-down that allows you to protect your fetus by sniffing out good and bad foods and surroundings. It's a fun experience if your newfound superpower doesn't cause you duress, but what to do if the scent of lobster bisque or your mother's perfume make you want to hurl? That's easy: Follow your nose. Avoid the offending aromas and foods whenever possible, and when all else fails, hurl away.

> "Try to get fresh air, sleep with the window open, and stay cool."

Snoring

The same swelling of the nasal passages that can cause the occasional nosebleed is also responsible for making you sound about as peaceful as a stuffed-up pug when you sleep. On the bright side, this symptom is definitely temporary, provided you weren't cutting wood in your slumber before you got pregnant. What to do in the meantime?

Give your partner earplugs. Sleep is very important right now. If you're worried about waking others you can deprive yourself of much needed R&R.

See remedies for Nosebleeds on page 104.

Ask your practitioner about sleep apnea. No need to get paranoid, but occasionally snoring can signify a condition that stops you from breathing for a few seconds during slumber. Since optimal oxygen is ideal for you and your wee one, chat with your doctor about your particular style of snoring.

Spider Veins

If you've got a little purple or red scribble patch just beneath the skin of your thigh, tummy, or face, you're the proud owner of spider veins, also known as "spider nevi" or "telangiectasis." Caused by capillaries giving in to the pressure from all of that pregnancy blood pumping through your veins, it can be quite pronounced during the duration, but should become barely noticeable after you give birth. Any remnants can be eliminated by a dermatologist. Still, there are ways to lessen the chance of getting or exacerbating them.

Don't cross your legs. It impedes circulation and can potentially encourage them.

Try natural remedies. Ask your practitioner about natural creams that may help, but don't try anything without a pro's go-ahead.

Stress

Relax and check out "Anxiety" on page 90.

Stretch Marks

Sorry, sister, the plain fact is there is nothing you can do to prevent stretch marks. Either you'll get them or you won't, and the decision-making factor has more to do with genetics than any fancy creams or balms you slather over your rubber band of a body. Miraculously, just like my mother, I did not get them—despite the fact that my boobs alone went from small handfuls to Dolly Parton contenders. However, I was not left unscathed. A year and a half after my daughter was born my skin still doesn't have the taut, youthful character of my bygone body. After being stretched like a blown-up balloon, my birthday suit hangs on my body just a little bit looser, as though I lent it to an elephant who squeezed into it and returned it a wee bit roomier. Additionally, various parts of my body—my breasts in particular—have become a walking example of gravity. (Of course some of my mommy friends don't have this same saga, so don't go wringing your bloated hands over it.)

There is an upside to the baggy look, however. Motherhood is the great ego-equalizer. Before being a mother I was acutely aware of my tiniest physical imperfections, from the skin tag on my eyelid to the few liver spots on my hands. From the day my daughter was born I couldn't care less about them or the new brown spots on my face, sagging skin on my knees, pooch on my previously flat tummy, or spider veins on my inner thigh. Life under my own self-critical microscope is over forever. And you know what? I'll take the liberating gift of self-acceptance over a tight bod any day.

Stuffy Nose

See "Congestion" on page 94.

Swollen and Sore Breasts

See "Breasts, Tender and Swollen" on page 93.

Swollen Hands, Ankles, and Feet (aka Edema)

Yes, you have turned into a human balloon. Only your hands, feet, and everything in between are not filling with air or even necessarily fat (although hopefully there's some of that since it's your body's way of saving up nutrients for the baby). The culprits are good old water retention, a regular and unthreatening pregnancy symptom, and blood volume, which increases by about 40% throughout this ordeal. As you near the end of pregnancy you may not be able to avoid parading around like an inflatable-float version of yourself. But there are some tricks you can try to stop yourself from looking like you deserve a prime spot in New York City's Easter Parade. Check them out and remember: Do not take herbal or other diuretics or any pharmaceuticals for swelling.

Watch your diet. For me this notion was futile. But if the discomfort and unattractiveness of bloating trumps your desire to overindulge at the breakfast buffet, here's to you! Try to eat high-protein foods such as chicken, fish, meat, cheese, and tofu. Also, see if high-potassium snacks, such as bananas, potatoes, or beets, help out.

Drink lots of water. Keep flushing your system by drinking at least eight glasses of water per day.

Drink warm lemon water. A warm mug of H_2O with lemon juice is refreshing for its taste and its ability to escort extra fluid out of your system.

Get a leg up. My most swell pregnancy experience happened at the five-month mark when I spent an entire day walking around New York City. By the late afternoon, I looked down and my ankles had literally disappeared. They had been replaced with mushy flesh that expanded to meet the width of my calves and left me with two stumps that had the shapeliness of elephant legs, minus the tan. Fortunately, they didn't stay that way; by the next morning my clubfeet were back to normal. But it was then and there that I understood why it's highly recommended to avoid standing for lengthy periods and to elevate your legs higher than your heart several times a day; it helps redistribute the water and blood to your upper regions. Should you choose to lie down, try to rest on one side rather than flat on your back, which can put pressure on major veins that carry blood to and from your heart to your feet and legs. (Not life threatening, but not ideal either.)

Watch for Sudden Swelling

Swelling and edema is a common and unthreatening pregnancy side effect. But after the 20th week, the sudden swelling of the hands, feet, and face in conjunction with elevated blood pressure and weight gain, and possibly headache, blurred vision, and seizures, can be a serious condition called preclampsia. Also known as toxemia or Pregnancy Induced Hypertension (PIH), it should be treated by a physician immediately.

Don't cross your legs. The look may be sexy, but you won't think so once you see the results of it stymieing your circulation. Sitting this way is also said to increase the possibility of varicose veins. Keep both legs slightly elevated—and uncrossed—whenever possible.

Exercise. Helping all of that blood to get pumping through even gentle exercise, like a nice stroll, can reduce swelling—provided you don't embark on an eight-hour jaunt through New York City.

Submerge yourself. Become one with your extra water weight. Take a body-temperature bath and submerge yourself up to your shoulders or go swimming; both will help your blood vessels reabsorb the freewheeling fluids.

Ask your care provider about supplements. He or she may recommend vitamin B, evening primrose, or magnesium.

Wear support hose. Many mommies turn to support hose to stop swelling. Ask your insurance company if they'll ante up before paying yourself; you might get lucky.

Urinary Leakage

See "Urination, Frequent, and Urine Leakage" below.

Urination, Frequent, and Urine Leakage

One of the weirdest parts of pregnancy for me was that I had to pee all the time during the first trimester. In the third trimester it made more sense; after all, I had become quite the water addict and there was a human bowling ball bouncing on my bladder. But how could one wily little sperm wreak so much havoc within the first few weeks? The answer is simple. You are producing more bodily fluids, your hormones are having their way with you, and later in the game your growing uterus is pressuring your bladder—literally. In the middle of pregnancy, as the uterus moves upward in your body, you may get a reprieve. (I did.) But in the third trimester don't be surprised if bathroom visits are back with a vengeance and a sneeze, cough, or hearty guffaw results in a subterranean sprinkle, if you know what I mean. But there is sunshine after the rain; these symptoms will disappear after you deliver.

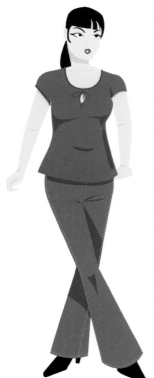

Keep drinking water! Don't let regular restroom dashes deter you. Drinking water is good for you and your baby, and potty pit stops are excellent ways to take breaks from your daily grind. Because I was working in an office with bathrooms that were very far away from my desk, I also considered my restroom treks a brief form of exercise and opportunity to break away from my computer.

When nature calls, answer. Pee as frequently as your body commands.

Do Kegel exercises. These exercises combat surprise sprinkles by strengthening the muscles around your vagina. They can be clandestinely done anywhere—from the privacy of your home to a seat in the boardroom. Here's what you do: Squeeze the muscles around your yoo-hoo as though you are trying to stop peeing midstream, pause for a few seconds, then relax. Do sets of 10 at least three times a day.

Wear mini-pads. If incontinence is an issue, minipads can catch you in the act and save you from having to repeatedly change your panties or pants.

Vaginal Discharge

With all those hormones bubbling around in your body, it's no surprise your yoo-hoo has something to say about it. Unfortunately, the conversation does not tend to be very polite. In fact, the farther along you get, it can contain unsavory words like runny, thick, smelly, heavy, and downright funky. What's a girl to do? Go with the flow, of course—and consider the following aids.

Keep it clean. It's a no-brainer, but now is not the time for a bathing hiatus. That said, douching is a serious pregnancy no-no, so stick to surface sprucing.

Let your yoo-hoo breathe. Forget fancy lace undies. Breathable cotton is your best friend now.

"Avoid standing for lengthy periods and elevate your legs."

Wear panty liners. Or at least keep them on you at all times. When needed they can save you from sloshing through the day. Change them regularly to keep your fanny fresh.

Keep an eye out for unusual colors and strong aromas. It may be hard to tell the difference between "normal" pregnancy goo and that of an infection, but if your nether region is itchy, odorous, or making particularly colorful (think green or yellow) or chunky deposits onto your panties, it's time to saddle up in the doctor's office stirrups and find out what's going on in there. Yeast infections are very common during pregnancy, and take it from someone who knows: without immediate treatment they can make sitting on hot coals seem like a comforting notion. At the end of pregnancy your discharge may suddenly sport a brown tint, which usually indicates the beginning of the breakdown of the mucus plug (a nice little blockade between the opening of your uterus and the rest of the world) and, consequently, labor. Pay attention and chat with your practitioner immediately if anything seems strange or you see any red or brown spotting.

Varicose Veins

The bane of many mothers, these unsightly swollen bluish stripes, which most often appear on calves and thighs but can also flare up on your vulva or anus (heard of hemorrhoids? See page 99), are essentially a plumbing problem. With up to 40% more blood flowing through your veins, it's quite a bit of extra work for the petite pipes of your lower extremities to fight gravity and push that extra volume back toward your heart. If their valves can't keep up, voila! You've got varicose veins. They are often hereditary and may be irritating, but they're not harmful and usually depart before or after you lose your baby weight. How do you handle them in the meantime? Read on. (Also see "Spider Veins" on page 106.)

Improve your circulation. It's exercise to the rescue again. Try the most inoffensive heart-rate raisers— walking or swimming.

Dress for success. Skip supersnug tights, pants, and especially knee-high socks, which can reduce circulation. Instead, check out support hose, which can help especially if you put them on before you get out of bed. (FYI, some insurance companies will sport for support hose; ask yours before blowing your hard-earned dough.) Also sport comfy, supportive shoes.

Take a stand or a seat. If you tend to be on your feet for most of the day, take sitting breaks. If you're prone to being on your

Braxton-Hicks

Braxton-Hicks contractions are warm-ups for the headline act. They can happen as early as 20 weeks into gestation and become more frequent the closer you get to your delivery date. If they occur more than four per hour, are accompanied by pain, or just freak you out, call your practitioner. Just how likely are you to get them? If the Mommy Menagerie's experience is any indication, you can consider these odds: Out of 97 women, 65% got them.

The Mommy Menagerie's Top 10 Creepiest Elements of Pregnancy

If you truly get that there's no sense in worrying about if or when any or all of these things will happen to you, read on. If not, spare yourself the anxiety and visit this section toward the end of your pregnancy when you can look back and laugh.

1. Vaginal Discharge
The #1 gross-out is the aroma, texture, and sheer volume of flowing goo that regularly lands on your underwear.

2. Alien Invasion
Even if it is your own kid, there is something pretty weird about having an individual camping out inside of you.

3. Scary-olas!
Nicknamed by a member of the Mommy Menagerie, the larger and darker areolas were right up there on the list.

4. Protruding Belly Button
Like a cooking thermostat that pops out when your meat is done, your "inny" belly button is likely to become an "outy" a few weeks before your tot is ready to pop.

5. Baby Acrobatics
As wonderful as it is, the feeling of a person moving around inside ranks as one of the weirdest pregnancy wonders.

6. Bloat of Arms (and Legs, Feet, and Face…)
It wasn't just the upper limbs, but the frightfully swollen feet and ankles that truly disturbed many of the mommies.

7. Tag, You're It!
Skin tags, or tiny little pieces of new skin, are just one of the fun new additions you are likely to find while searching the newly foreign land that is your body.

butt, get up and walk regularly—including when you travel.

Don't cross your legs. It decreases circulation.

Elevate your legs. Relax and prop your legs up above the level of your heart multiple times each day. Also, while sitting, prop your feet up on a stool.

Vulvar Varicose Veins

See "Varicose Veins," on page 109, for suggested actions.

Yeast Infections

My most annoying pregnancy predicament was definitely the run-of-the-mill yeast infection, partially because I got them continually and also because I could never tell whether monilia (yeast) was again hosting a party in my puhana or whether my Chinese-torture-like drip was amniotic fluid. It was this confusion that had me racing to my doctor's office a number of times late in the pregnancy, waiting to be told that childbirth was imminent. But again and again it was just a beloved yeast infection. It gave a whole new meaning to a bun in the oven. Is it possible to avoid yeast infections if you're prone to them? Got me. But here are ways to try.

Take the advice offered under "Vaginal Discharge," page 108.

Air Things Out. Go light and breezy by sporting skirts.

Eat Yogurt. They won't cure a raging infection, but yogurt's cultures help increase your system's helpful bacteria, which can help with prevention. For a fab yogurt recipe, check out page 62.

Get a prescription. My doctor said Gyne-Lotrimin and Monistat were pregnancy-appropriate aids, but don't take her word for it. Ask your practitioner which medicines are safest for you.

8. Leaky Faucet

What's not to love about the occasional urinary leakage? According to the Mommy Menagerie, plenty.

9. Hey, Big Mama!

A bulging midsection didn't surprise the mommies, but the supersizing of the vagina was another story altogether.

10. Stretch Marks the Spot

You really may just earn your stripes during pregnancy.

Pregnancy At Its Worst

Here's something that should make you feel a lot less fearful of childbirth: out of 108 mothers, only one of them mentioned contractions as one of the worst physical side effects of pregnancy. So, what topped the Mommy Menagerie charts? Following are a list of common complaints and the percentage of women who weighed in on them.

Lower back pain or sciatica
21% of women felt back ailments and "SY-attic-a" were two of their greatest woes.

Nausea or morning sickness
For 16% of mommies, the desire to hurl was the sickest pregnancy element.

Swelling and bloating
A whopping 14% came in with complaints of Fred Flintstone feet, cankles, bloating, or swelling of the hands, feet, and lower legs.

Sleeping sagas
7% deemed discomfort or difficulty in sleeping an eye-opening dilemma.

Weight gain, exhaustion, hemorrhoids, or hip or pelvic pressure
With 6% of the vote each, it was a four-way tie for these maddening maladies.

Leg cramps, constipation, indigestion/heartburn, or restless leg syndrome
According to 4% of women, these four possibilities felt even less fun than they sound.

Gas, stretch marks, varicose veins, or leg and feet aches and pains
3% sounded off on these four pregnancy follies.

Carpal tunnel syndrome, foot growth, huge boobs, acne, hernia, chaffing, or anxiety
Each of these captures the hearts and minds of 2% of the voting population.

Singular sensations
What was most miserable to 1% of the mommies? Of the 108 mommies who answered the question, there was one vote each for Vulvar varicose veins, intolerance to hot weather, feeling ugly, itchy breasts, general discomfort, and congestion.

The Mommy Menagerie's Creepiest Moments—In Their Own Words

If you're looking for a heads-up on some of the funky fun that might be heading your way, here's your chance to read some highlights of the Mommy Menagerie's answers to the question, "What was the creepiest physical element of pregnancy?"

"All the discharge (that no one told me about!) and just how big the vagina gets. My god."

"Bloody noses and needing to spit a lot; basically becoming a human mucous factory."

"The first time my breasts leaked freaked me out. It was the colostrom, but when it happened it looked like slime."

"Vomiting so hard it came out my nose is about the grossest thing that happened to me. It took two years before I could eat yogurt again."

"I had major urinary leakage problems for about half of my pregnancy. The first time I 'wet my pants' I called the doctor thinking my water broke. I wore a panty liner for four months. It totally sucked."

"The worst one was every time I threw up, the force of the pressure on my stomach would make me pee. I always had to change all of my clothes. It was not pretty."

"Honestly, it was good creepy, but the feeling that another being was rolling around, flipping, contorting itself in my abdomen felt really weird sometimes."

"The first times I saw an elbow or foot poking my belly from the inside."

"Top three would be: You grow a new organ! (The placenta.) I thought that was quite creepy. . . . The stretching of my belly skin—who knew it could go out that far? And those big blue veins that showed up all over my new large boobs. They looked like some kind of ugly road map."

"The skin on my back and my chin broke out badly. My underarms also got much darker."

"My hair began to grow really fast and thick—everywhere!"

"Right around three or four months I got the worse case of pimples on my shoulders. I had about 50 pimples on each shoulder. I had no idea that would happen. They lasted about two weeks then went away."

"The dark line down from navel to vagina, and dark spots on my face that never went away."

"Dark large areolas . . . yikes. . . . Not very pretty to catch a glimpse of in the mirror!"

"All my moles on my neck quadrupled in size because of the growth hormone in my body. They all went back to normal afterwards, but it still was creepy."

"Just seeing the body expand and wondering if it would ever go back to normal. But it was kind of cool, too."

"Watching my boobs morph into two gigantic melons that individually were bigger than my baby's head when he was born. I was totally horrified."

"Round ligament pain was weird. I could tell that something was going on down there and sometimes there were stabs of pain or like a stitch in my gut."

"The way my ankles looked. They swelled up so much
that they were practically nonexistent. . . . Also, the
skin on my ankles and legs was a weird consistency. If I
pressed the bloated ankles and lower legs with my fingertips, they would stay indented like Play Doh."

"My varicose veins in my vulva!!!!!!!!!!!!!!!!!!!!!!!!!!!!!!!!"

"The varicose veins that seemed to be popping up at an
alarming rate! Also, I got all these broken capillaries on
my face and chest. The amazing thing is they went away."

"In the third trimester while having sex my vagina felt sort
of swollen internally, like it was a much tighter fit for my
husband, and could be a little uncomfortable. It was like
feeling internally congested. Oh, and skin tags, mostly
around my armpits. I hate those things."

"It was creepy to have sex and feel the baby moving
around at the same time. It was also creepy after the baby
was born and my breasts would squirt milk during sex."

"I thought the whole mucus plug thing was rather
strange. . . . I lost mine bit by bit and the consistency was
so alien to me, and I never knew if it meant it was 'time'
or what? Of course, when it finally dislodged before I
went into actual labor, there was no mistaking it for the
real thing. It was like a glob of blood-streaked slime."

"The worst element by far of pregnancy was post-partum.
I have never felt so awful for so long in my whole life. I
breezed through pregnancy and had the delivery experience I wanted. I thought I was through the worst of everything until I hit post-partum, which lasted far longer than
I ever thought. Also, no one feels sympathetic towards you
anymore since you are no longer pregnant!"

Despite a two-week debilitating back problem, occasional sciatica, and recurring yeast infections that were so itchy that sitting on a hairbrush was a tempting form of relief, I felt great throughout most of my pregnancy—physically. The psychological side of the scale was not as tilted in my favor. Though I am generally a pretty perky gal and remained jubilant for most of the pregnant duration, I had some Empire State Building-like hurdles to clear during the three trimesters—sometimes while dragging weight that amounted to a couple of Thanksgiving turkeys attached to my tummy, thighs, and chest.

Early on I battled spontaneous hormonal combustions where I felt extreme laugh-out-loud glee, tear-inducing grief, and teeth-clenching anger all within the course of a minute—during a simple radio commercial. Throughout the entire pregnancy I waddled through rivers of sadness since my husband was not yet onboard with being a daddy. From five months on I shouldered the stresses of managing the editorial department of an Internet startup, moonlighting as a freelance writer, and planning an elaborate post-elopement wedding party. Toward the end I suffered from the "Oh-my-god-I've-blown-up-like-Violet-Beauregard-in-Charlie-and-the-Chocolate-Factory" syndrome. Only rather than a rotund purple-hued figure with tasty gum, I had blotchy skin and cottage-cheese thighs.

Still, I had a fabulous time. How? During the physically and mentally trying times—and also in the times in between—the second best thing to having a sense of humor and reminding myself that everything was temporary was to pamper myself—regularly and unabashedly. I spend quality time with friends, pets, and my belly, watched movies and went on dates with the hubby, got massages and pedicures, ate yummy food, lounged, and treated myself to lip glosses and eyebrow waxes. And when sadness or anger occasionally became overwhelming, I wholeheartedly indulged myself in those, too!

Of course you don't need drama, pain, or depression to pamper yourself silly. You already have the perfect excuse: You deserve it. And besides, your baby definitely benefits from your feel-good vibes (and equally feels it when you stress).

The Art of Pampering

To me, "pampering" is anything you do specifically to take care of and treat yourself in a special way that goes beyond the everyday. A pampering gesture can be as simple as a breath of fresh air or a soothing bath, as elaborate as a spa weekend or a shopping spree. It can range from a guiltless fruit smoothie or a shameless piece of triple chocolate cake. It can cost nothing but a few free moments, or enough to make your credit card company place your account on hold.

In the throes of morning sickness, exhaustion, forgetfulness, and the awkward experience of the ever-expanding body, even the most proactive pregnant woman can forget to pamper herself—not to mention how to do it. If you need a little schooling or just a few fun ideas on how to perk up your day, flip through the following pages for heart-tickling treats, Mommy Menagerie favorites, and—when times get really tough—ways to help you forget for a moment that you're a human zeppelin on stumpy bloated stilts.

Indulgence doesn't have to be expensive or time consuming. The following efforts are easy to integrate into your regular routine.

Show how much you care.

If you're feeling down, overwhelmed, underappreciated, exhausted, scared, or just plain ugly, give yourself a call and leave an affirming message on your voicemail. Or write yourself a love note and pop it in the mail.

It may sound goofy, but this fun trick has surprisingly uplifting results.

Besides, everyone likes to be told they're beautiful, loveable, fabulous, strong, exceptional, and special—and there's no better messenger to help internalize your self-confidence than you.

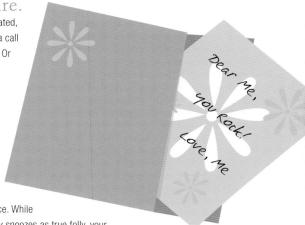

Dear Me,
you rock!
Love, Me

Take a nap.

This is one indulgence you should seriously embrace. While your pre-pregnancy self may have looked at midday snoozes as true folly, your new body-built-for-two actually needs extra rest. Don't be afraid to take it—whenever and wherever you need it. If your boss finds you curled up under your desk, I'm sure he or she will understand. (Not.)

"Write yourself a note and pop it in the mail."

Do nothing!

That's right. You now officially have permission to loll, recline, idle, dillydally, and lollygag. So what are you waiting for? The next time you feel the urge to alphabetize your CD collection, plow through that imposing stack of bills, or calculate how to finance you child's education, instead take a pause, plop onto the couch, and relax. All of your must-dos will still be waiting for you tomorrow, and once your new addition arrives, the list will be never-ending.

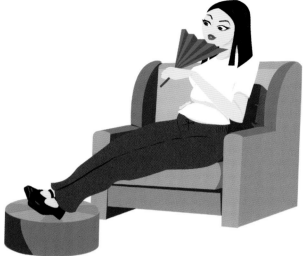

Take a bath.

Indulging in a warm dip has dual benefits: Soaking is a very relaxing experience, and it stops you from doing little more than reading or chatting on the phone. Later in pregnancy it's also kind of fun to see your island of a tummy peeking out above the bubbles.

Take a walk.

Such a simple and accessible pleasure, yet often overlooked, going for a walk can clear your head, invigorate your spirit, and count as a bit of exercise—a recommended activity that generally results in feeling groovy.

Spend time with your pet.

This may sound crazy, but as a bona fide cat lady who had two teenage Siamese cats when I gave birth, I can tell you that your relationship with even the most beloved pet, if you have one, will never be the same after you have a baby—not even close. It is a sad, but true fact that there just isn't time and energy to love and attend to your baby and Fluffy or Fido with the same gusto of yesteryear. Plus, it won't take long for your four-legged favorite to figure out he or she no longer rules the roost. You'll see for yourself soon enough. But meanwhile, take my word for it and consider special time with your pets a fantastic indulgence that should be exploited to the fullest while you have the luxury.

Visit with friends.

Hanging out and gossiping about everyday things may not fall into your "indulgence" category now, but trust me: Once your world revolves around diapers, naps, and burping, they will be as easy to come by as a free vacation to Hawaii. Take time to savor your friendships and the freedom to indulge in them. While they won't completely disappear once your bundle of joy arrives, they are likely to be put on the back burner for quite some time—unless you've got nearby family that lives for babysitting or Madonna's nanny budget, and enough stamina to dance on the bar on a Friday night and run a marathon the next morning.

Get a makeover at a cosmetic counter.

This is one of my favorite indulgences even when I'm not pregnant. After all, what's not to like about having someone fawn over you, tell you that you look fabulous, and pull out all the cosmetic tricks that make all of those celebrities look better than they do in real life. Best of all, it's free—provided you can resist purchasing all of the powders, creams, and pencils that have made you feel like a pregnant Cinderella the night of the ball.

Take pregnant portraits.

You can't beat your growing body (and definitely shouldn't try), so why not join it by celebrating your new shape. Take plenty of pictures that accentuate your motherly figure (ideally naked) and make sure to note when the photo was taken. Even if you're not feeling so fabulous now, after the fact you will wish you had evidence of your internal adventure.

Write in a journal.

Penning the details of your pregnant life does more than chronicle your experience, which, by the way, you will definitely forget once the baby comes. It allows you private time, quiet concentration, and the opportunity to vent, celebrate, dream, and rant to your heart's content. If you ask me, it's the cheapest form of therapy. Next time you're feeling wound up about something, try writing down the whole saga and see if the anxiety leaps out of your head and onto the paper. Another fun thing to note is your impression of your fetus's personality. Is he or she feisty or languid? Playful or shy? Pen your impressions now and revisit them after he or she is born. You may be surprised to see just how much your kid's character was showing itself before it was born.

Pregnancy Portrait Tips

Primp beforehand, act like you think you're sexy and fabulous when taking the photo, and set up the shot in front of an attractive backdrop. I had my husband take some snapshots, but foolishly thought of it more as a quick, unplanned documentation than posed portraiture. In my naked pregnancy memento, I'm unceremoniously standing in front of a funky unlit fireplace with my panties at my feet, a bed-head hairstyle, makeup-less face, and a Post-It with the date scribbled on it stuck to my thigh. Every time I look at it it's not my wildly rotund figure (which in retrospect looked surprisingly good), but my underwear, unkempt hair, and uneven skin that stops me from feeling a sense of pride and accomplishment.

INEXPENSIVE EFFORTS

If you're the type who has a hard time blowing money on unnecessary items, here's a fact that may just make you feel better about dipping into your fun-funds for small treats over the next nine months: Once your baby is born you are likely to stay home a lot more for the first two years—and as a result spend a lot less money on yourself.

Give yourself flowers.

My husband does lots of things to show he cares, but unless it's my birthday or the very occasional surprise, gifting me with a beautiful bouquet isn't one of them. If you need a little pick-me-up, don't wait for someone else to lift your spirits. Buy yourself a bunch of Gerbera daisies, elegant calla lilies, or commanding dahlias; snatch up a perky mixed bouquet or a blooming potted plant from the grocery store; or order a stunning arrangement and have it delivered—with a gushing, flattering note about how great you are, of course! Place your aromatic artwork on your desk at work or bedside table at home so it will continually brighten your day.

Go to the movies.

You've probably heard it a gazillion times by now: Get your fill of your favorite outings—movies, dinner, whatever—now because it'll be much harder once the baby comes. Whether you are with company or going it alone, take a load off your body and your mind by watching an upbeat movie at a movie theater. (Downer movies aren't conducive to pampering.) If you tend to get uncomfortable sitting for long periods of time, bring a couple of pillows—one for your butt and one for your lower back. Don't forget the bonbons and kick up your feet if you can. Now that's living.

Eat something delicious.

Great food is a treat even when you're not pregnant, so it's no surprise that the Mommy Menagerie ranked it highly when asked the best way to pamper the weary mom-to-be. Top on their list was ever-popular ice cream ("And not the low-fat stuff either!"). Next up was the simple notion of forgetting about dieting and instead eating with a carefree attitude. Going to restaurants also made the list—and was one of my personal favorites. Should you treat yourself, you know better than I just what would hit the spot, but if you need some inspiration, check out Chapter 3, where you'll find fast and delicious pregnancy-craving recipes by some of the nation's top mommy and daddy chefs.

> "It's amazing what a sprinkle of glittery shimmer can do to brighten spirits."

Buy beauty products.

It's amazing what a dab of color, sprinkle of glittery shimmer, or swipe of high-gloss lip sheen can do to brighten sullen spirits. For a fast pick-me-up, drop by a drugstore, boutique, or department store and scan the cosmetics area for makeup and accessories that are whimsical, feminine, and a little more playful than your everyday choices. Purchasing a new shade of lipstick, some body glitter, sparkle nail polish, or luxurious hair products and cute accessories every now and then helped me to focus not on the giant blob I had become, but on one single supercute thing about me: glittery toenails, my newly thick hair pulled back with a pretty clip, or how great I smelled thanks to morning applications of In Fiore body balm made by my very talented friend Julie.

Get a manicure, pedicure, or both.

The pedicure was the Mommy Menagerie's number-one way to indulge. Why? For one mom, it was the chairs with back massagers. For another, toenail tinting was a fun outing for her and her four-year-old daughter. For me, it was the combination of sitting down, catching up on the latest trashy magazines, getting a foot massage, and primping the only part of my body (other than my hands) that looked like the old me. Glistening, shaped, and prettily poilshed toes were my beacon of glamour and civility amidst a sea of very unglamorous and rogue body experiences. FYI, it freaked me out to sit and sniff the fumes that came with neighboring acrylic nail applications, so I usually asked to sit near the door and that it be kept open. If you're inspired, do the same, or skip the salon altogether and hold your own nail-painting party at home—with friends or just your fabulous self.

Go on a date with your partner.
Scooting out to a movie, dinner, or round of mini golf will soon be a special occasion. Seize these moments and savor playtime with your partner as much as you can while the world revolves around just the two of you.

SPECIAL TREATS
Desperate times call for desperate measures. When life is really getting you down or you simply need something to transport you from your busy everyday state of mind into a few glorious moments of pregnancy nirvana, try any of the following activities—as often as you can.

Play hooky.
Who cares if you're taking off on maternity leave soon, have loads of housework, or a cranky kid at home. Every now and then it's important to revitalize yourself and the best way to do that is to make space for all-about-you time. Call in sick, put off the housework, or hire a babysitter if needed. Then do something completely and utterly self-indulgent. If you feel guilty about it consider this: You're much better at your job, being a mother, sweet wife, and overall decent human being when you give yourself time to relax and regroup.

Get a facial.
As much as I enjoy having an esthetician slather products all over my face, I almost never get facials because if I'm going to splurge on spa treatments I can never pass up a massage. But if your skin is wreaking havoc on your self-esteem, a facial does double-duty as a relaxing treat and a complexion enhancer, so long as you go to a trustworthy place that understands the pregnant skin dilemma.

Get your hair done.
Yes, there are two schools of thought on pregnancy and haircuts. I've heard people say never to get a cut while pregnant. Others, including a handful of women from the Mommy Menagerie, see an hour in the chair and under the dryer as a form of heaven. I'm somewhere in between. Pregnancy may not be the best time to embark on a completely new and adventurous hairstyle—especially a short one that makes your plump face look like a full moon—but it's a fantastic time to celebrate and revel in your mane, especially since it is one thing that is sure to look really fabulous while you're pregnant. (You usually lose hundreds of strands of hair per day, but while pregnant your body holds onto it, so your hair is bound to look thick and luminous.) I made a final trip to the salon just before giving birth and was very glad I did; I didn't return to the chair for nearly a year—when my thick pregnancy hair abandoned ship and I was suddenly in desperate need.

In any case, keep in mind that a bad haircut could stymie an already unstable sense of self-esteem, so stick with colors and cuts that you know you like.

Go clothes shopping!

This preferred pick-me-up of the Mommy Menagerie can be a delightful excursion or a slippery slope, depending on where you are on the pregnancy timeline, how you're feeling about yourself when you go, whether you foolishly torture yourself by going to stores that won't have anything that could possibly fit you, and how much self-restraint you have when you see the perfect maternity T-shirt for $100.

If you're like me, you'll hold off on shopping until the last minute, when you're feeling so down on your looks and desperate for change that you'd almost consider selling your car for a complete fashion makeover. My advice to you is don't wait until you get to that point. It's like going grocery shopping when you're really hungry; you always grab

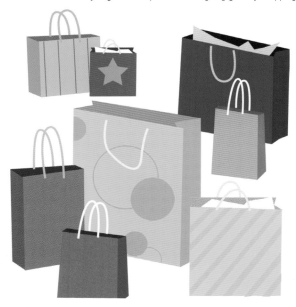

impractical junk that you'd normally pass up for more sensible options. Regardless, there is no denying the power of garments that make you feel good about yourself, which explains why you just may end up spending more than any rational woman would on clothes that are likely to fit you for less than a year.

If you're going to hit the stores, take my advice: Avoid shops that don't have clothes that will fit you; they are really, really depressing. If no such store exists, head to an accessories boutique where one size really does fit all. You can also shop for Baby, which is always fun. But to avoid buying stuff you'll never use, see the tips in Chapter 14, page 224. And for good sources for pregnancy fashion, shopping, and all things retail, see Chapter 13.

Get a massage.

For many Mommy Menagerie members, this pricey treat was worth the splurge, especially when it included a good prenatal massage therapist and special bed padding that allows a mommy-to-be to safely lie on her stomach or sides without discomfort or strain. While this hands-on outing outranked every treat but the pedi, it was not a slam dunk; one mom couldn't truly relax while her baby kicked around and the other found the positioning, pillow propping, and changing of positions uncomfortable. Should you be inclined, seek a licensed therapist who is trained in pregnancy massage and knows to avoid aromatherapy oils and potential contraction-inducing pressure points in the hands and feet.

I definitely indulged in massage during pregnancy, but unfortunately it was by force when my back went out and I was in desperate need of pain relief. Were I to do it all again, I wouldn't wait for more of an excuse than this one: Whether pregnant or not, massage causes me to slow down and relax and makes me feel very, very good.

Get a wax.

I never got to the point where I couldn't see my feet, but my bikini area did become a foreign land visible only by a glance in a full-length mirror. Not that I cared. My husband wasn't embarking on any adventures down under, so to speak, and unlike some women I really didn't feel a need to impress my delivery doctor with a perfectly preened yoo-hoo. Nonetheless, waxing is another easy way to treat yourself to something that makes you feel like the old you—and look a tad sexier in your maternity underwear.

For me brow waxes had huge benefits that could be appreciated by all. The day before I went into labor I got them done and really did feel wonderfully pretty because of it. (And oh-how-shapely and fabulous they must have looked when they practically jumped off of my face at the first signs of intense labor pains.)

SERIOUS SPLURGES

While shopping for clothes and baby stuff could certainly fall into the category of serious splurges, the following treats are more likely to create memories that last well beyond the dent in your credit card.

Partake in a girlfriend weekend.

You may not want to go to Vegas and dance on the bar all night, but a special getaway with your gal pals is incredibly rejuvenating and fun, whether it's a spa, ranch, river retreat, or girlfriend's house. Even more important, it's an opportunity to spend focused quality time with friends that you may not see much of for the first several months after the baby comes. (And after that, unless they're also parents, you may not have a lot in common to talk about anyway.)

The Mommy Menagerie On .... Pampering Pleasures

"I ate out a lot instead of cooking. That was pampering to me."

"I watched a lot of 'Sex and the City' on DVD."

"My normally clear skin went crazy during pregnancy, so I treated myself to a montly facial. It really helped."

"I had a semi-regular massage. I would recommend that highly. It was hard to find the time, but it really helped me mellow out."

The Mommy Menagerie's Pampering by Numbers

The Mommy Menagerie's top ways to treat themselves while pregnant are ranked by popularity and listed in percentages of women who mentioned the indulgences as preferred pampering. They will hopefully inspire you. Take it from women who know: Do it now, often, and whole-heartedly; the opportunities down the road will be few and far between—and if you have another baby you won't have the luxury of free time while in waiting.

38% preferred pedicures.

36% were fans of massage.

12% favored food.

12% turned to rests or a nap.

9% sent themselves shopping.

8% got merry on manicures.

8% benefited from baths.

7% didn't pamper themselves.

7% had their hair cut or styled.

5% were fond of facials.

5% loved body lotions, oils, scrubs, and butters.

5% turned to the TV or movie screen.

Embark on a babymoon.

Another worthy excursion that cannot be stressed enough, the babymoon is a structured opportunity to spend quality time with just the two of you, provided you have a partner and actually want to spend extra time with him or her. While you may not fully grasp just how all-consuming having a baby is just yet, believe me when I tell you that you will never ever ever have a life that is about just the two of you again. Now, that's not a bad thing. It's the reason you got pregnant, after all. But it is also a real reason to celebrate, honor, appreciate, indulge in, and savor the special bond that you share. Spending time together now will give you goodwill reserves to help you get through the sleepless nights, baby vomit in your hair, fights based on nothing but exhaustion, and every other fun twist and turn that you will face together.

Travel!

Before I had my daughter I thought I could just give birth and continue my life of adventure. I was wrong. It's not that I couldn't travel with a baby. Before she was eight months she'd already been to New York twice, Hawaii, South Carolina, and Los Angeles. But after a year it became clear that it was far easier and more relaxing for everyone if we just stayed home for the time being.

Plainly put, it's just not as much fun to travel with a baby, especially if you are aware of and sensitive to his or her needs (and of course you will be!). So, if you've got the travel bug, indulge it now, ideally in your second trimester when you are feeling your best and still mobile enough to hoof it without too much exhaustion. If you want to go international, check with your doctor about any required shots or precautions.

Regardless of where and when you go, bring a copy of your medical records in case you need to visit an out-of-town hospital.

Let friends and family throw baby showers for you.

Now this was one of my very favorite indulgences: a great party that's all about you, for you, and not thrown by you! In my mind there are no rules when it comes to baby showers for first-time mommies—except that guests shower you with attention and great baby gear. You can have one party or ten. They can be thrown by family or friends, and can be all women, all men, or a mix of both. It can be a daytime party or an evening event. The only words of wisdom I can give you is that if you really want your guests to give you items from your baby registry, make sure that the host stresses that to the guests.

When my shower was thrown for me I put off buying most of the essentials, expecting that they would be plucked from my baby registry and delivered to my door. But it turned out that most of my guests—especially those without children—either didn't check my registry or didn't want to give a practical gift. Almost everyone was—and is—a sucker for cute baby clothes. So, instead of a diaper bin, bibs, and zip-up PJs with feet, I got an adorable and very tiny Viva Las Vegas tank top, an array of zero- to three-month outfits that my child never wore since I was too afraid to manhandle her little limbs and rubbery neck early on and preferred to stick her in easy PJs, and enough onesies that my child would never have to wear the same one twice. For a list of what I consider must-haves, see Chapter 14, page 209.

I'd been running and lifting weights five days a week on a regular basis when I peeked at the pregnancy stick. At the time I felt fortunate that my body was strong, fit, and prepared to pull its own weight and then some, and I continued to do some form of exercise—mostly walking and weights—well into the third trimester. (That's when trucking to and from the office became more than enough of a workout and the ideal fitness regime consisted of hoisting myself up to the couch, getting horizontal, and exercising my right to do absolutely nothing.)

But nine months down the road, there was nothing fun about comparing the snapshots of the old bikini-clad me to the new wide-angle whale who could pummel the bygone Gidget with one swing of an Amazonian breast. In short, exercising didn't stop me from becoming a house. But perhaps it did help me to transition into a cute little condo rather than a sprawling ranch. I am certain it helped me to stay strong, energized, and upbeat, not to mention confident that the old me existed beneath the layers of lard.

I found out a year and a half and many trips to the gym later that this was indeed the case. While pregnancy definitely changed my body forever (my boobs are bigger and my "problem areas" have shifted, for example), exercising has minimized the impact and helped me to rebound physically and emotionally.

"your body will thank you for busting a stretching move."

THE BENEFITS OF BREAKING A SWEAT

I've always been a physical person and have long appreciated the self-confidence, heightened energy level, and euphoria that come with working out, so it seemed perfectly logical to me to continue exercising throughout all three trimesters. However, today's paranoid and decidedly delicate view of pregnancy can make even the most active mommy-to-be fear that a simple morning jog might run that little fetus right out of your yoo-hoo. If you fall into the fearful camp, it may be soothing to know that according to virtually all current medical sources, including top pregnancy resource The American College of Obstetricians and Gynecologists, nothing could be further from the truth.

Now may not be the time to take up boxing, football, snowboarding, or other intense new sports. But creating or continuing some kind of exercise regime can dramatically improve everything from your state of mind to the state of your behind. Still married to the couch? Consider all of the perks: According to The American College of Obstetricians and Gynecologists, exercising now will increase your energy level; relieve constipation, leg cramps, bloating, and swelling; lift spirits; help you relax; improve your posture and quality of sleep; promote muscle tone; control gestational diabetes, fight back pain, give you the extra stamina and strength to help with labor and delivery; and possibly even shorten and ease the efforts of getting your Mini Me out into the world. Need more reason? How's sheer vanity? A little athletic investment now will give you a head start in getting back in shape after the birth.

What more do you need to know, other than forgiving and comfy yoga pants may quickly become your new best friend? Read on for fitness facts, tips on how to ease pregnancy pains, and plenty of encouragement to work it out.

If you're already active:

Most doctors agree that there is no need to immediately change your routine just because you're baby bound. In fact, current wisdom suggests you go ahead and do your thing, provided your pregnancy is not considered high-risk, you do not introduce new highly strenuous activity into your regime, and you are not a hard-core athlete such as a professional skier or marathon runner. (In the latter case, you should discuss the safety of your routine with your practitioner.)

If at some point your morning jog just doesn't feel right anymore, modify your workout. For me, the transition from unabashed athletic pursuits to more guarded aerobic gestures (brisk walks, light weights, and stretching), came at three months. But everyone is different, as was evidenced by a woman in my prenatal yoga class who effortlessly

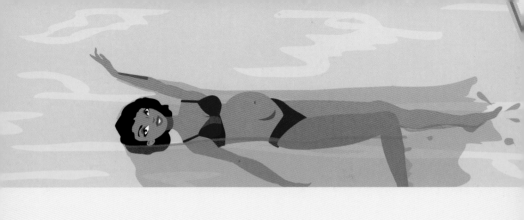

catapulted her lithe body into a handstand at nine months. (Had I tried that, my girth would have succumbed to gravity and buried my head into its own folds.) As with everything else in pregnancy, the key is to trust your gut—and avoid doing anything that you might attribute as a cause if anything goes wrong.

Even if you're happy with your current regime you may want to explore pursuits that are especially good for the pregnant body, and are preventative and preparatory for childbirth and beyond. Read on for details.

Just for beginners:

If you haven't been exercising in the past, your current inclination may be more along the lines of lounging on the couch than lunging toward the gym. But as you settle into pregnancy and start putting on the pounds, your body will thank you for busting a stretching and strengthening move.

How do you get started? Choose a program you like that is safe for your body. The American College of Obstetricians and Gynecologists says almost any form of exercise is safe if it is done with caution and you don't do too much of it. (A few sports are not recommended; see the "Exercise No-Nos Cheat Sheet" on page 134 for details.)

Swimming, walking, and cycling are excellent and very safe aerobic options, while basic pregnancy stretches and prenatal yoga classes with a trained professional can help ease achy muscles and minds and strengthen areas that are bearing your baby brunt.

THE EXERCISE BASICS

Regardless of whether your idea of exercise has been lifting the TV remote control or running half-marathons, you can benefit by knowing the essential ins and outs of pregnancy exercise listed below.

Be mindful of your health status.

High-risk pregnancies or other factors such as heart disease, vaginal bleeding, potential preterm labor, multiples pregnancy, preeclampsia, and ruptured membranes, are good reasons to ensure you're set to sweat. If you have any concerns about exercising and your health, talk it out with a professional beforehand.

Find good ways to work it out.

The key to a great workout routine is doing something you enjoy. Walking, swimming, bike riding, jogging (only if you were already a runner before you got knocked up), low-impact aerobics, pilates, yoga, weight training (with pro supervision), and chasing after your other children, if you have them, are generally considered fine practices for perspiration. If you're feeling really spunky, mix up your routine to keep things exciting.

Stretch.

It is always important to stretch before and after you work out, but it is especially important while your body is under invasion. For recommended websites that address the subject, see Sources on page 242.

Tread carefully.

Before you unabashedly dash out onto the hiking trail or even to the grocery store, remind yourself that your body is not its old self. The same hormones that allow your svelte cervix to make way for a human watermelon causes other joints to stretch and become more loosy-goosy, too. As a result, carelessly bounding about can cause injury. Additionally, all that weight focused on your front stresses the lower back and pelvis and can cause instability. So, look at yourself this way: You are now a Weeble with the wobble but not the "won't fall down" guarantee. Exercise— and move through daily life—accordingly.

Monitor your heart rate.

Those extra pounds will ultimately increase your heart rate and consequently cause some huffing and puffing while you're standing still, never mind strolling on a treadmill. While the old adage was to ensure your heart rate doesn't top 140 beats per minute (which mine does anytime I step on the treadmill, pregnant or not), lots of professionals are now recommending a more flexible means of monitoring yourself: Whenever you step up your activity make sure you can talk normally without gasping for air. It'll ensure your body is getting enough oxygen to all the right places, including your internal air-conditioned condo (aka uterus).

Dress for success.

Now's not the time to slack on supportive shoes or bras. I went on a tri-city treasure hunt to find a sports bra that could comfortably harness my heretic chest. But finding a sling that adequately strapped down those jugs made the difference between wincing with the slightest bounce and prancing as freely as a braless pre-teen.

Dressing in layers is also important, since heat and humidity easily overheats and melts the warmly wrapped mommy-to-be when she cannot strip down to lighter garb.

Hydrate.

If you don't want to steam like an engine without coolant, keep water nearby and gulp it down regularly.

Practice Those Kegels!

Kegel exercises, which work out the pelvic muscles and prepare them for pushing out a tot, are recommended for even the laziest women in waiting. And they can be done without getting off of the couch! For details on how to do them, see page 108.

Trust your body.

If you feel more like exercising your right to lie on the couch than to take a hike, go with your flow. Since flexing and stretching your muscles is bound to give you more physical and emotional energy, it's not the best idea to completely give in to pregnancy laziness. But on the days that you feel too tired to exercise, don't. Your body is the boss now, so do what it says.

Don't sweat the fat stuff.

Unless you're one of those pregnant women who looks like a model with a basketball tucked under her shirt, there is likely to come a time when you won't be too pleased with your full-body profile—especially when standing next to those ubiquitous gym or jogging path nymphs who flit around in a Spandex second skin. My remedy for this: Don't look! When you catch a glimpse of yourself in the mirror, wave and move on or focus on something pleasant about yourself like your thick hair, gleaming eyes, or fresh mani. It also never hurts to follow the heavyset herd to a prenatal exercise class where you are likely to see women who are faring better and worse than you.

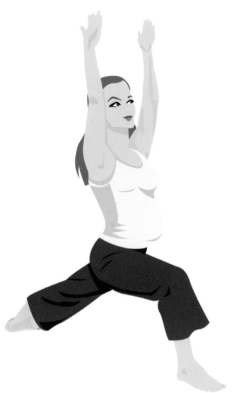

10 Commandments of Pregnancy Exercise

There is no one right way to exercise during pregnancy. But there are a handful of tenets worth warding.

1. Talk with your practitioner about suitable exercise.

2. Aim for 30 minutes of activity several times per week.

3. Stretch before and afterward.

4. Be careful.

5. Hydrate.

6. Dress for success.

7. Follow your body's cues.

8. Don't focus on your fat.

9. Stop the second something doesn't feel right.

10. Remember that the goal is never to lose weight.

Mommy Menagerie's
Top 10 Favorite Exercises

Check out the physical activites that kept 111 mommies moving.

1. Walking
59% enjoyed hoofing it on the treadmill or elsewhere.

2. Yoga or prenatal yoga
32% considered doing the downward dog an optimal exercise experience.

3. Doing absolutely nothing from the get-go or early on
16% preferred to take it easy based on everyday habits, how their body was feeling, or doctor's orders.

4. Swimming
11% put their maternity suits on and took to the water.

5. Chasing toddlers around
10% considered tending to their tots more than enough exercise.

6. Bike riding (outdoor/stationary/recumbent/spin classes), running, or jogging
9% put the pregnant pedal to the metal or enjoyed trotting their unborn tot around.

7. Water aerobics, water walking, or weight training
6% of mommies turned to water movements or weight lifting.

8. Elliptical machine or Stairmaster
4% preferred the aerobic activities of gliding or stair climbing.

9. Hiking or Pilates
3% of mommies headed for the hills or Pilates classes.

10. Everything else
1% of the menagerie opted for one or more of the following for exercise: bar-method strength training, cross training, gentle stretching, hip-hop class, toning and strengthening class, gardening, excessive house cleaning, or working on your feet all day.

The Mommy Menagerie On ...Exercise

"I couldn't exercise in the beginning (sickness) and then I just gave up. I walked the stairs, but that was it."

"I wasn't allowed to exercise per the doctor's instructions. (I can't imagine I would have wanted to anyway!) I did walk the dog and hoped it burned more calories than my normal state sitting at the computer!"

"Exercise? Where would I find the strength? Lol."

"I did not exercise during my pregnancy, mostly because I did not exercise before my pregnancy. My husband and I were in the habit of taking walks in the evenings and I continued to do this to the end of the pregnancy. I took pre-natal yoga classes and swam a few times. Both of these activities came in the last trimester."

"I didn't really do much because I work all the time. I tried to buy pregnancy workout CDs but they bored me. I even went so far as buying a gym-grade elliptical trainer, which I used a total of 12 times. I would dissuade pregnant women from buying gym equipment since another friend of mine also bought a treadmill and rowing machine (also barely touched). I surrendered at the end of the seventh month and took to indulging in reading a novel a week. I decided to exercise my mind and let my body relax."

"I got a Pilates DVD, but I'm pretty sure it still has the plastic wrap on it."

"I walked a minimum of two miles pretty much every day up until I delivered the babe. It wasn't just my exercise, but my stress-reliever too."

"My mother-in-law came to live with us unexpectedly when I was four months pregnant. She had dementia and 'low-grade' Alzheimer's. My walks were my salvation for blood sugars, stress-relief, and bonding time with my dog."

"Not much other than walking (and yoga in the first month), because I was afraid that I had done too much exercise before my miscarriage. Starting in my seventh month I went back to yoga classes."

"Walked regularly till last trimester, then laid around like a beached whale."

"I stopped working out at the gym after the first three months. Just walked after that. Started walking a lot during the last month to try and get things moving."

"I started out exercising, but then was put on bed rest for a month during my first trimester because my son was sitting on my cervix. Because it was my first pregnancy, I was totally freaked out and afraid to exercise after that."

"I walked during my first trimester, but by my 25th week I was no longer allowed to do even that because of contractions, so I ended up having a very sedentary pregnancy. I felt guilty about it, mainly because everyone I know is such an exercise nut. In my heart of hearts, I was glad to have a legitimate, doctor-ordered excuse to be a couch potato."

Exercise No-Nos Cheat Sheet

First, it's important to ask your practitioner if you have any health conditions that might limit your active pursuits. Second, it's not recommended to start any strenuous new exercise regime without consulting your practitioner.

 Skip the following exercises:

Deep knee bends or lunges. They can strain ligaments and possibly increase the chance of tearing the pelvic region. Youch!

Full sit ups. After the first trimester these are no-nos because the position pressures a major blood vessel and impairs blood flow to your brain and uterus. Besides, consider this fun-creepy fact: abdominal muscles often divide down the middle during pregnancy and part like a curtain to make way for your star of the show. Pressuring them doesn't help matters. (Yes, they reunite after the fact.)

Double leg lifts (lifting and lowering both of your tree trunks simultaneously). Ditto above.

Straight leg-toe touches. Once you can't see your toes it's a non-issue, but until then forgo the forward fold. It could injure the tissues connecting your back joints and legs.

Exercises after the first trimester that require you to lie on your back. Again, they can block blood flow to the brain and uterus.

 Forgo activities that require great balance or have significant crash-and-burn risks. Specifically:

All contact sports. Bedroom athletics aside, slamming into other people isn't advised.

Downhill skiing. It's not the skiing but the falling that makes hitting the powder a no-no, although hitting moguls certainly can't promise a smooth ride for your baby-to-be.

Gymnastics. Ever seen a pregnant gymnast? Enough said.

High-impact aerobics. Even if your joints welcomed the jarring motions, your newly flexed ligaments and potential instability make low-impact the way to go.

Horseback riding. Sorry, sister. The only stirrups you should be straddling right now are the ones in your doctor's office.

Ice skating. Your body's being taxed enough. Why risk slamming it onto the cold, hard ice?

Inline skating. Gliding's great, but your loose ligaments may not agree. Better to spin your wheels some other way.

Jogging on rough terrain. The risk of becoming a human tumbleweed is too great.

Racquet sports. Combine jerky motions, freshly flexible joints, and unfamiliar weight distribution and you're courting serious potential for strains and topples. However, some sources say playing doubles (triples if you count your prenatal partner) is safe since you don't have to cover as much ground.

Scuba diving. Morning sickness is bad enough. The last thing you or your fetus want is decompression sickness—and rumor is that a fetus can get it without mommy even knowing.

Snowboarding. If you've ever caught an edge you know darn well why you should not strap on your boots and board and hit the mountain.

Surfing. Half of the sport of surfing is falling (at least if you're me). Last time I checked, no doctor has recommended headers as positive pregnancy activities. Besides, putting your weight onto your rounded tummy to paddle out seems just plain wrong.

Waterskiing. One minute you're up, the next minute you're down—with an involuntary enema and the occasional body slam as unexpected bonuses. Better to wave coyly from the boat.

 Remember the rule of thumb: Don't do anything that feels risky to you or that you would blame if something goes wrong.

 Don't exercise in super hot or humid weather.

 Do not continue if you begin to suffer from any of the following: Dizziness, faintness, shortness of breath, rapid or uneven heart beat, chest pain, headache, vaginal bleeding, uterine contractions that continue after rest, subterranean leakage, discomfort, or decreased fetal movement. If you're remotely concerned about an exercise experience, contact your provider ASAP.

My husband actually thought I was following one of my kooky whims when I announced one Sunday morning that we should stop by the drugstore to get a pregnancy test. An hour later he stood in the bathroom doorway, slack-jawed, as I jumped up and down waving the saturated stick with such elation that I didn't realize the extent of my husband's horror. (In his defense, we had only known each other for six months.) From then on we had two very different pregnancies.

Mine overflowed with excitement, curiosity about every little detail, and optimism about a new future together. I read books, scoped out baby clothes, researched classes, wrote a book proposal for this book, talked about it all the time . . . and prodded him to be equally enthusiastic.

His was anxious, distant, and full of dread. He gnashed his teeth over all the guys at work who told him life as he knew it was over, stopped trying to feel the baby kick because I invariably put his hand on my belly too late (early on it's like trying to point out a shooting star), and internalized his anxieties about the present and future.

Rationalizing that he was entitled to his own pregnancy experience, I tried to focus on the positive—and found it regularly in little things, like the way he excitedly bounded out of the doctor's office during the amnio because he couldn't wait to call his parents and tell them we were having a girl. Or when he came home from a trip and presented me with a Dallas Cowboys pacifier and bib. Or, later in the pregnancy, when he and our unborn daughter started playing "knock-knock" with each other on my belly.

If you asked Colie about pregnancy today he'd tell you that he didn't like it. He felt alienated and very disconnected from the experience, and that frustrated him. I've heard of women whose husbands were extremely into pregnancy—sometimes even more so than the mommy-to-be. But if you're partner is in more of the bah-humbug or "Oh s*#t!" camp, let me tell you something that may boost your spirits: The minute our daughter arrived, Colie couldn't have been more into her. As a new daddy, he could finally relate to something tangible and he's been cooing, coddling, and fawning ever since.

Transitioning to a Threesome

Many partners don't feel particularly connected to pregnancy or understand that you have new needs that must be addressed. And given that the party is all going on inside your body, it's no wonder. They don't sense the queasiness that arises from a whiff of lobster bisque, experience the intense internal changes (though surely many of them revel in the expanding bust line), or feel inclined to disown family members for eating the last bowl of cereal. And from what I've heard from mommy friends, they generally aren't reading pregnancy books to help enlighten them. Unless they are pregnant or have been pregnant, it's impossible for partners to wrap their heads around the new you. In fact, they may not truly grasp that their pregnant partner is indeed changing until there is physical evidence in the form of a midsection metamorphosis—and I'm not just talking big breasts; I mean a full-blown basketball tummy.

Plainly put, you're having a very intimate and exclusive new relationship with someone else while your partner stands on the sidelines without the faintest idea of what's really going on—other than perhaps that he (or she) is now supposed to be supportive in some new and different way. For some couples, navigating the nuances of this new threesome is as effortless as sailing along with a blowing afternoon breeze. But for others it can be as strenuous as trying to go against the flow without a mast—without the proper steering equipment, there's no knowing whether you'll crash onto the rocks or sail into the sunset. Should you feel as though your relationship has been cast into the wind without solid direction, read on for perspective, understanding, and communication tools to help turn the tides.

Honing Your Communication Skills

Communication is the key to any great relationship, but it becomes even more imperative when you become a walking bag of unpredictable pregnancy hormones, are experiencing the elations and anxieties of a major life change, and are developing new, unexpected, or inexplicable needs and desires. Rather than waiting for the shiitake to hit the fan, better to brush up on your communications skills beforehand. Here's how:

Ask for what you want and negotiate when necessary.

You may know that the ice cream in the freezer is off limits, the baby's room absolutely must get painted this instant even though she's not expected for months, and that a compliment goes a long way in quelling your insecurity around your newly rotund figure. But the people in your life are not mind readers. Without adequate communication, they may have absolutely no understanding of your needs or desires and fall into a trap of failed expectations around finishing off the Rocky Road, watching the game while using the unopened paint can as a footstool, or affectionately calling you Thunder Thighs.

In the world of relationship communication, no request is too great or too small, especially during pregnancy, when you may need or want things that are unexpected or unusual. Does requesting what you want guarantee that your partner will happily dash off at 3am to satisfy your sudden need for peanut butter? Not necessarily. But at a minimum it will give your partner a better understanding of where you are emotionally. Ideally, it will also open a dialogue for sharing feelings and negotiating. A wise therapist once advised me that in relationships it's ideal for both parties to ask for 100% of what they want 100% of the time and negotiate from there. If you want the room painted and your partner wants to watch the game, a fair negotiation might be that the nursery will get a fresh coat of pale

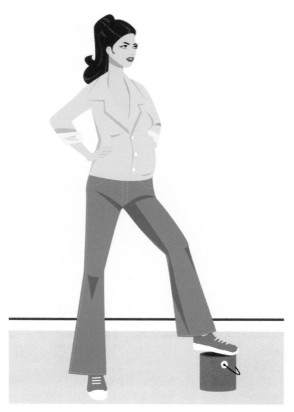

pink right after the ninth inning. With that knowledge you can relax and focus on something else—like when he or she is going to dash out for that peanut butter. Or if negotiations clarify that your needs are not going to get met by the person in question, it's in your best interest to instead turn to someone who is willing to help. (See "Build a good support system" on page 141.)

Make sure your expectations are mutually agreed upon.

The surest way for people to fail your expectations is to assign the expectations to them without their knowledge or agreement. When my husband and I first started living together, I would get really mad at him when he didn't take out the trash the minute it was full. I figured that since I did the shopping, cooking, and cleaning it was the least he could do, so when he came home exhausted from work and carelessly stepped over the pile of recyclables gathering at the base of the garbage can, my blood boiled. But in retrospect the fault really resided with me. Though I had asked him to take out the trash on a number of occasions we never had a real discussion and agreement about who owned garbage duty and exactly what that would entail. Once we had that conversation and agreed upon terms, we shared the same expectations and our garbage sagas went out with the trash.

If you find yourself getting pissed off that your loved ones aren't meeting your expectations, take a step back and evaluate whether they are aware of your expectations and have agreed to them. If not, revisit the tip on the previous page. But remember: just because you ask for something doesn't mean you'll get it. Negotiation and compromise are part of the deal, even for the pregnant woman.

Explain what is happening for you during moments of clarity.

Most of us reserve sharing our less savory sides for the people closest to us because we know they will still love us even if we act like a complete lunatic from time to time. If you dip into emotional darkness, lose your cool, or put loved ones through the emotional grinder more than usual during pregnancy, pause when you're wearing your maternal halo rather than your horns, and explain your situation and your need for support. Fair warning doesn't mean it's open

"The surest way for people to fail your expectations is to assign expectations to them without their knowledge."

Ask for What You Want

When asking for what you want, the more specific you are the better, especially if you are likely to explode if you don't get exactly what you had in mind. If there is a margin for error, outline the details in writing. This is an especially good exercise when it comes to grocery shopping.

season on those closest to you, but hopefully it can help them be especially understanding and supportive during this time of hormonal heresy.

When I started going into labor at three in the afternoon in mid-August, I called my husband at work and calmly told him it was time to come home. His job was an hour away from our house in Napa Valley, California, and the hospital was in San Francisco, a good hour drive, too. (No, I was not worried about getting to the hospital in time—from all of the labor stories I'd heard, it'd be a miracle if that baby was speedy enough to pop out on the same day, never mind as we made our way across the Golden Gate Bridge.) When he got home, we sat on the couch, watching TV and timing my painless contractions until they were an hour apart, which was when the hospital recommended we get in the car and start heading to town.

Over the course of the pregnancy my occasional emotional explosions had not been well received by my other half, so it was not without trepidation that I felt one coming on as we headed for the door. It wasn't anything in particular that set me off. I just suddenly felt oversensitive—to my husband's voice, to the songs on the radio, to, well, everything. But this time I handled it differently—or to be more specific, I handled it in a way that benefited both of us. Rather than opening my mouth and vomiting my annoyance all over my unsuspecting husband, I calmly said, "Look, honey. I'm starting to feel oversensitive to everything right now, and I want to ask you a big favor. Whatever happens from here on out, can you take absolutely nothing personally and let everything roll off your back?" He agreed and later told me how helpful that cue had been to him. Prepared and on the same page, he didn't freak out when during labor I screamed "No!" when he touched me, or barked at him when he attempted to coach my breathing despite the fact that seconds later I obediently followed the very same advice from a nurse.

Because I communicated my needs in a way that could be understood by my husband I got what I needed in a way I hadn't before.

Ask for clarity rather than making assumptions.

Even people who are excited about the imminent addition may not show enthusiasm the way their pregnant partner wants them to. Rather than deciding what he or she thinks or feels, it's always a good idea to get firsthand information straight from the source.

This advice would have been especially handy for me during my last trimester when my husband and I attended childbirth and newborn classes, each of which were broken up into three evening courses. Along with preparing us, I saw them as opportunities to get Colie more excited and educated about the pregnancy in a way that my blathering and the unread stack of books I had piled on him had not seemed to achieve.

Unaware of my expectations, he approached the first session with class clownery that I usually adore. He drew a turtlehead at the base of a spinal cord diagram in our workbook, juggled the plastic baby while learning to change diapers, and doodled head-down while the instructor led discussions and demonstrations. All the while I sat silently, fuming, having decided that he was not taking the class and our pregnancy seriously. At home that night I exploded, and went to bed sobbing.

Colie did not fool around during future classes, but to have that be the end of the story would be missing the point. Freaking out on him may have stopped him from joking, but it did not get at what I really wanted, which was to know that he cared and was paying attention. In retrospect, I could have pulled him aside at the time and said, "When you draw instead of watch the teacher I make myself think that you aren't paying attention, don't care, and will not be prepared to help me when I go into labor. Is that the case and, if not, would you mind reassuring me?" Had I done that, perhaps he would have reassured me that, despite his chiding, he was indeed interested and absorbing the information. (I learned this was in fact the case when he reiterated coaching instructions word for word weeks later when I went into labor.) Or maybe he would have shared his own feelings about the experience—his apprehension, fear, confidence, or excitement. But I'll never know because I didn't ask.

While having the clarity to reach out for a reality check in the midst of an emotional eruption is about as likely as fitting into your skinny jeans in your ninth month, it's worth trying to keep it in mind. Checking in for your partner's perspective instead of deciding for yourself what's happening is healthy for your relationship in general, and becomes even more handy when you and your partner are sleepless and trying to navigate life with an ever-needy newborn.

> "Checking in for your partner's perspective is healthy for your relationship."

Make honey-do lists.

It's not unusual for the pregnant woman to suddenly get a fierce nesting instinct, inspiring her to embark on major home-improvement projects, purchase every baby room item necessary, and clean the most intimidating closets and drawers in the wee hours of the morning.

While partners tend to be along for the dust-busting ride whether they like it or not, I found that mine was more receptive to a written list of tasks rather than one that was barked at him in no particular order and with no end in sight. Unlike women, who are natural multitaskers, men work best when they focus on one goal at a time. Give a guy a prioritized list, or better yet, discuss the notion of setting up a Dry-Erase board and dividing tasks under headlines of "Urgent," "1 week," and "ASAP." If he agrees to work from it, you may find that your tasks get done without argument and your man actually gets excited about adding feathers to his nesting cap.

Build a good support system.

One of my greater pregnancy mistakes was expecting my husband to attempt to make everything better when I was feeling blue, needy, or downright crazy. Why? First, while he has many fantastic traits, the art of comforting isn't high on the list. Second, he felt very excluded from the internal mother-child interaction and consequently wasn't into the pregnancy. Third, he couldn't relate to being pregnant. Yet I craved empathetic girlfriend-y conversation, coddling, and motherly love from him.

It finally occurred to me that it wasn't necessary or practical to attempt to get all of my needs met by him or any one person. We all look to different people in our lives to satisfy different needs. I rely on a writer friend when I need computer advice, a mom of three for parenting insight, and a chef pal for culinary queries. I would never expect the childless chef to clue me in on the secrets of breastfeeding, nor would I expect the mom of three to know the best online source for round wonton wrappers. So why expect that my stoic, kitchen-challenged husband cheer me up by whipping up a fantastic dinner and begging to hear every emotional and physical nuance of my day? When it became clear that no amount of cajoling would turn my husband into a girlfriend (which, incidentally, I am very happy for), I expanded my support system so that in times of need I could run through my mental rolodex and turn to the person with the best skill set to address the needy woman at hand.

I'm sure some pregnant women are surrounded by partners who do everything necessary to make them happy. If you're one of them, lucky you. For the rest of us, the point is, there's no sense in trying to force people in your life to be something they're not. If you yearn to compare and share your ailments, empathize about your body's ever-changing state of anarchy, chat about the perfect nursery furniture, or anything else that doesn't come

TO DO:
- ☑ take out trash
- ☐ assemble crib
- ☐ give partner massage
- ☐ buy groceries

The Mommy Menagerie On
...Feeling Supported by Your Partner

101 mommies weighed in on whether they felt supported.
65% said yes.
15% said no.
18% found middle ground.

Want some explanations? Read on.

"Yes, but I actually wished he'd done more for me, like get me pedicures. I wanted to feel like someone else was pampering me and though I never directly said, 'I want you to pamper me by getting me pedicures,' I said it in front of my partner to many male friends who asked for advice. My husband never picked up and did anything with that. Perhaps if we have a second, he will. Or I'll just tell him this time."

"Yes, although I felt that there were some things he just could not understand—like the need to eat, NOW."

"Pretty much, maybe sometimes I wanted a little more acknowledgment that carrying a baby is a big deal and can be uncomfortable; how about a massage?"

"Yes, although it's hard in the beginning when you don't 'look pregnant' yet. They don't get that you're really feeling pregnant even though you don't look like it yet."

"Mostly. The exception was when I was having trouble breast-feeding and he couldn't comprehend why I couldn't just make it work."

"Yes. . . . other than him thinking I could still do everything physically that I did before, like carrying laundry up and down stairs and moving the couch to vacuum."

"As much as a man can understand why you are crying one moment and happy the next."

"No, he thought I would puke or gag loudly to get attention. He was sympathetic, but begrudgingly. We would have fights where he would say that he wanted me to be nicer. I guess I was just supposed to be jolly about throwing up every other hour throughout the day."

"No, I talked to my girlfriends about what was going on with my pregnancy."

"No. He just panicked so I had to spend a lot of time reassuring him that it would all work out. The second time around he has been very supportive and excited, with only a few moments of worry."

"No. I tried to talk to him about it, but ended up really being supported by other women, friends, and relatives who have been there before me."

"No. I threw a few tantrums myself to get my point across, which didn't really work. Then I started a Log of Complaints to get his attention in a humorous way with entries like, 'Asked subject if he could put lotion on my back because it is itchy. Said he is busy and will be there in a sec. Fifteen minutes later and subject is still in front of his computer text messaging.' Whenever he refused a pregnancy request or wasn't supporting me in the way I needed, I would read entries from the journal and we would both laugh. Later when he saw me pull out my journal, he would drop what he was doing."

"One thing I expected from him that I never got—and frankly, didn't ask for—were foot rubs, back rubs, massages, and just general physical support. I didn't want to have to ask for these, which was ridiculous in hindsight."

naturally to your partner, seek support elsewhere. Outlets can be as free-form as phone calls to friends, Internet chat rooms, or online bulletin boards (see Sources, page 238, for good options), or as structured as local support groups through medical, community, or baby centers. Whichever options you choose, they are bound to be more fruitful than expecting empathy from someone whose closest experience to pregnancy is overindulging at the all-you-can-eat buffet. An extended support system is also likely to ensure you get all of your emotional needs met and find more peace and appreciation for your partner.

Remind yourself that though you deserve

to be the center of the universe right now, you may not be. I have a theory that people generally think about others for about 15 seconds and then go back to thinking about themselves. This notion is fantastic for soothing yourself

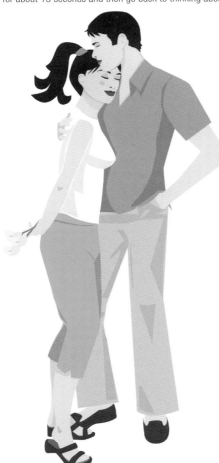

after you've said something really stupid at a dinner party or had a houseguest announce to your entire backyard picnic that their toddler just ransacked your bedroom and found extremely personal items. But it's also a helpful tip to remember throughout pregnancy. In the moment, it may seem like everyone around you should be able to appreciate and sympathize with your predicament—not to mention drop everything and beg on bended knee to be of service anytime you are in need. But it's likely that they are actually thinking about their own lives, occasionally recalling that you are perhaps not feeling or acting like yourself, and if you're lucky, pondering how to improve your day. This can especially be true for daddies-to-be who are going through their own pregnancy emotions while coping with yours.

For this reason, along with communicating your needs, feelings, and wants to those close to you, it's a good idea to reiterate them more than once if necessary and, when it's clear that your partner is just not up for meeting your needs, turn to others in your support system.

Praise your partner.

There's an undercurrent of uncertainty and excitement that goes along with pregnancy. There's also a lot of attention being put onto you. Turning the limelight onto your loved one every now and then by specifically outlining his or her fabulous traits or recent deeds is a healthy way to share the love, and get more of the good stuff sent your way. In other words, remind your partner of how wonderful, supportive, and special he or she is—often.

In fact, praising your partner can be a good way to offer suggestive hints as well. Take, for example, my friend who loves to get flowers but hated the bouquets her boyfriend regularly gave her. Not the supermarket-mixed-selection type of girl, she saw his offhanded offerings as statements that he didn't understand her

Read Aloud to Share Important Information

If your partner isn't into pregnancy books, but you feel some information within them may be helpful for your partner to know, read passages aloud. I can't tell you how many times I said something like, "Hey honey, this book says that I should get massages regularly after the first trimester to help my back," or "This article says, my mood swings are the result of biochemical change in my body that is real and that I cannot easily control." Sometimes I was fishing for sympathy, other times I was trying to prepare him. But in both cases, telling him the information I wanted him to know helped me to feel better, whether he was interested or not.

style and taste. She wasn't foolish enough to lambaste him for giving her a gift; she knew it really was the thought that counted and that a lashing wasn't about to get her a fast floral encore. Still, she was hell-bent on getting her guy to show up holding either a bouquet of one type of flower sans garnish or a sculptural modern masterpiece. So what did she do? Praised him when he gave her the flowers, heralded the types of arrangements she likes when they encountered them out in the world, and wove in hints along the way. She'd look past the baby's breath and fern leaf filler of his latest bestowment and say, "Oh, thank you baby! I LOVE calla lilies. They're so simply festive they don't even need adornment! They look fantastic on their own in one big bunch."

A few months and hints later, he hit the botanical bulls-eye.

Sometimes straightforward talk is the way to go, but in the other instances, praising things that your partner is doing well, or that you want done a little differently, is a delicate way to direct the future.

Say thank you.

Late in pregnancy I felt it was my divine right to have everything I wanted—and, in many cases, that my husband had to get it for me—be it a hug, foot massage, glass of water, or command over the TV remote control (for all three trimesters and beyond). Why shouldn't I bark requests from the couch? After all, I was doing all the work! Whenever he kindly or reluctantly accommodated my whims—which was regularly—I made a point of clearly and sincerely expressing thanks and detailing the thoughtful things he had done for me. I knew that it was important to recognize his contribution, especially since much of the attention around the house was squarely focused on my big belly and me. Besides, no one likes to feel like a slave. A little appreciation goes a long way—and makes men feel helpful, which they tend to like very, very much.

Ask for your partner's perspective.

It's easy to get wrapped up in your own experience that you may forget that there's plenty going on for your partner, too. Keep communication channels open by checking in and getting a fresh view from the other side of the fence.

Remember that your partner isn't you.

As much as you may want your partner to have the same pregnancy experience as you, it's not going to happen. Just because you're the one carrying the baby doesn't erase the fact that he or she is bound to have his or her own interest level, emotions, thoughts, fears, elations, and reactions to the pregnancy. These facts can be particularly frustrating if you're dying to pontificate on the nuances of pregnancy while your partner would rather watch sports highlights, the stack of pregnancy books left for him or her gathers dust, or your craziness is met with defensiveness or retreat rather than open arms. If you're feeling frustrated with your partner's lack of understanding or participation, try to remind yourself that the behavior doesn't necessarily translate to disinterest. Everyone has their own way of coping and adjusting, and for many partners of pregnant women, parenthood starts when the baby is born.

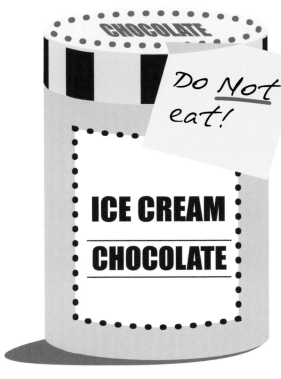

If you and your partner are not on the same philosophical or emotional page now, consider it a great opportunity to fine-tune the art of agreeing to disagree in a healthy, productive way. This is a tool that will become essential the minute you have your first (inevitable) opposing view of child rearing.

"As much as you may want your partner to have the same pregnancy experience as you, it's not going to happen."

10 Tips for the Pregnant Woman's Partner

Hand this section right over to your other half:
Greetings! No need to read an entire pregnancy book to know the secrets on
how to keep a pregnant woman happy. Heed these 10 tips and you're golden.

1. Do something nice for her every day. A shoulder massage, affectionate snuggle, bouquet
of flowers, gift certificate to a spa, love note, compliment, anything you know that
makes her feel special.

2. Feed her! When she says she needs a cheeseburger now, she means RIGHT NOW. You
cannot begin to understand how dire the situation is for her, but you can avoid her wrath
with a quick response.

3. Don't be late! Or if you are behind schedule, call ASAP and let her know. If you are
bringing dinner home, forget calling and consider promptness a matter of life and death.

4. Don't eat anything that isn't known as common property—and if you want to be on
the safe side, don't finish off the last of anything in the fridge or cupboard; in case of
emergency make sure your pregnant partner knows about it before she is ripping
everything out of the cupboards searching for it.

5. Don't take any crazy behavior personally or hold it against her. Instead, give her space,
offer a hug, or ask her if there's anything you can do for her. This isn't only a kind
gesture, but also a good maneuver for self-preservation. Resistance is futile.

6. Don't tell your wife she looks large—ever. If she asks if she looks fat and the answer
is yes, lie, lie, and lie again.

7. Understand that even if she seems fine, she's not feeling remotely normal. She's likely
to get crazy-tired, crazy-hungry, and crazy-sensitive so try to be understanding if she
doesn't rise to the usual occasions.

8. Never disagree with a pregnant woman—she is always right, even when she's not.

9. The bigger she gets, the more frequent the compliments. It's hard not to feel insecure
when your figure goes horizontal. Show your appreciation for her shapely sacrifice by
telling her how beautiful she is—regularly.

10. Help her when she's huge. Nothing comes easily when you're packing on that much
poundage, including getting off of the couch or out of bed.

Extra: Give her a token of appreciation after the birth. Soon you'll know the real meaning
of hard labor. Acknowledge her achievement with a special gift. Skip flowers—
everyone will send them. Go directly to jewelry—engraved with a sweet
sentiment. She'll never forget your thoughtfulness.

The Mommy Menagerie On
...Was your partner into pregnancy?

111 mommies shared details on how their partner responded to their new status.

81% of mommies said their partners were indeed into it.
5% said their other half was not.
14% landed somewhere in between.

Read on for further explanation.

"Yes, although it's hard in the beginning when you don't 'look pregnant' yet. They don't get that you're really feeling pregnant even though you don't look like it yet."

"Yes. But definitely more the second time around because he was totally freaked out the first time."

"He was happy I was pregnant, but he did not read books, ask questions, or talk to the baby."

"Does twisting his arm to get him to go to the 20-week ultrasound during our first pregnancy sound like he was into it? I almost let him skip out on the one-day labor class we took together since he found it to be quite ridiculous. . . . although he liked the Bill Cosby video at the end."

"Not as much as I would have liked. Sometimes it seemed more real to me than him. I had to keep reminding myself that he didn't live this day in and day out like I did."

"Yes, but I actually wished he'd done more for me, like get me pedicures. I wanted to feel like someone else was pampering me although I never directly said, 'I want you to pamper me by getting me pedicures.' Perhaps if we have a second, I'll just tell him this time."

"Sometimes too much."

"Yes, although I felt that there were some things he just could not understand— like the need to eat, NOW."

"Not until 22 weeks, when he saw it on ultrasound for the first time."

"Pretty much, maybe sometimes I wanted a little more acknowledgment that carrying a baby is a big deal and can be uncomfortable; how about a massage?"

"My partner was more into it than I was."

"Mostly. The exception was when I was having trouble breast-feeding and he couldn't comprehend why I couldn't just make it work."

"As much as a man can understand why you are crying one moment and happy the next."

The Magic Words Cheat Sheet

One day my husband asked me what, exactly, I wanted him to say when I was hitting an emotional wall. I told him that "I'm sorry—that really sucks" was the perfect response to pretty much any problem and that extra Brownie points would be gained by following up with, "Is there anything I can do for you right now?" Colie's said those very words ever since. He doesn't understand how reciting a script can be an effective form of consolation if we both know that it is a preplanned sentiment rather than a heartfelt response. My answer is simple: The mere fact that he says what he thinks I want to hear shows that he understands my situation and recognizes my need. At the end of the day, my husband's acknowledgment that I am in a dark place is comforting no matter what the day's dilemma. If the same could be true for you, see if your partner will try these phrases in an emotional pinch.

 How to Address Sadness or Anger
"I'm sorry—that really sucks."
Or
"Is there anything I can do for you right now?"
Or both.

 How to Address Image Issues
"You always look beautiful."
Or
"I've never seen you look more beautiful."
Or
"You are the most stunning pregnant woman I have ever seen."
Or
…You get the picture.
Even better is if your partner says this regularly, unsolicited. Every waddling woman can benefit from a little buttering up.

Let me first say that I was not fashionable throughout my entire pregnancy—and I was the executive editor of a fashion website at the time! Everything was fine while I could still force my way into my regular wardrobe, but the minute I had to bring on a bulge-chic look, I was completely lost. As a busy working girl I didn't have much time to research my choices, so when the day came that I truly couldn't wedge my way into my pants, I fled to San Francisco's maternity stores in a state of desperation.

First stop was Japanese Weekend, a Mommy Menagerie favorite. But everything there actually made my short stocky body look worse. I left crying. Next was Mimi Maternity, another Menagerie-preferred boutique featuring trendy fashions. But their selection had been picked over by more prompt pregnant shoppers. I had a little better luck at Old Navy, where I got two long-sleeve T-shirts and a pair of elastic-waist pants that I instantly had to return because they fell down every time I bent over.

By the time I stumbled into A Pea in the Pod, I would have traded my tagalong husband for a decent ensemble. Instead, I swapped next month's rent for anything and everything that seemed remotely attractive, even though the prices were higher than I would normally pay for things I could wear for years.

When buyer's remorse set in, I returned a few items, but I did keep key clothes that lasted for the long haul: great maternity jeans that fit until the final stretch and back again, a pair of black maternity Capri pants, a bra, a stretchy fitted black v-neck T-shirt with three-quarter-length sleeves and a slimming ruched front, two stylish everyday T-shirts, and one black dress.

I collected a few more pieces along the way—two maternity sweaters, two tank tops with built-in support, several bras, a gift of a maternity sweat suit, and two fabulous hand-me-down blouses. From there I integrated clothing I already had, such as cardigans (unbuttoned), loose skirts (hung low), a stretchy sundress (forever stretched beyond repair), my favorite pair of low-waist stretchy jeans (they finally ripped), and a pair of old cotton shorts.

At the end it wasn't pretty, but by the time I needed help tying my shoes and pulling up my panties, I couldn't have cared. Ease and comfort were all that mattered to me. Perhaps that will be the case for you, too, but if it's not, you're in luck because unlike me, you have the advice of more than 100 mommies on how to sashay through pregnancy in practical, comfy style.

WADDLE WITH SOME STYLE

From my perspective there is absolutely nothing worse about pregnancy than fashion. It's one thing to feel like a walking barf bag, bundle of raging hormones, or overstuffed sausage. But to feel like that on the inside and look just as miserable on the outside can be a real downer for even the most upbeat mommy-to-be—especially since beyond having to surrender your body, you may also sense your personal style going the way of your waistline. I'm here to tell you that needn't be the case—especially considering all of today's maternity wardrobe options.

More and more clothing companies are catering to the maternity shopper, but apparently many of them also know that there's little a pregnant woman won't do or pay for something—anything!—to make her look better and feel more comfortable. Thus, you might reach a point where spending $80 on a cute fitted T-shirt seems like a small price to pay for a little style sanity. But if you read these pages, you'll have more affordable escape routes should you choose not to blow your unborn child's college tuition on a wardrobe that you are guaranteed to despise in less than a year. Of course if you have that kind of money to spend, power to you, sister!

Regardless, this chapter offers myriad ways to feel and look at least somewhat like your old self as you waddle down life's runway, including practical guidelines for what to buy and what to avoid, Mommy Menagerie fashion tips, beauty basics, and lots and lots of empathy. Once you've got it dialed, flip to page 182 for shopping sources.

Before you start styling your newly grand girth, there are a handful of things you might want to know.

Comfort is key.

You may humor yourself at first by squeezing into your regular pants or cramming your cans into your everyday bra, but after even one bout of gut-wrenching gas or a painfully bouncy dash for the elevator, you'll realize that absolutely nothing takes precedence over comfort. In other words, if you've been known to buy clothing that looks better than it feels, think twice; that cute pair of jeans that makes your newly bigger bootie look perky at the store but cuts a wee bit at the waist is likely to live on the hanger once it gets home. And most maternity stores only offer credit, not cash refunds, so even one false purchase can have you cornered.

You will ruin your pre-pregnancy clothes

if you force yourself into them. At some point the only truly cooperative pieces of your old wardrobe may be your socks. But you can do damage long before then. Just ask my forever-stretched sweaters, pre-pregnancy bras, favorite jeans, and two pairs of flannel PJs, which ripped in the rear. If you care about your clothes, tuck them away until after you have your baby and are close to your pre-pregnancy weight. This goes for strappy sandals and other stretchable shoes, too, unless you're willing to toss them post-partum.

"There is absolutely nothing worse about pregnancy than fashion."

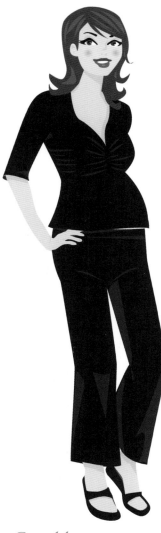

Fitted is more flattering.

The baggy look isn't becoming of anyone except supermodels who could benefit from the appearance of a little more meat on their bones. Besides, the pregnant body is most beautiful when heralded rather than hidden—even if your puffy perspective doesn't see things that way. Still, when buying maternity gear, it's a good idea to stay with stuff that isn't too tight. Instead select styles that gently hug your curves. As one Menagerie member put it, "Don't try to hide your shape. You'll end up looking like a tent with a head."

Black is the new slim.

The fact that wearing black makes you look more slender is not new news, but it is worth reiterating now that you're rocking the round look. The sophisticated color is also very versatile, so a pair of black maternity pants, a black shirt, or a black dress can be accessorized any number of ways for a variety of looks.

Stretchy fabrics rule!

You will soon discover that staying outfitted in great maternity clothes requires as much updating as keeping a baby fashionably dressed; what fits one day may be outgrown the next. While this is less true of forgiving maternity pants with superstretchy bellybands and T-shirts with ample elasticity, it is certainly the case for stiff shirts, fitted sweaters, and possibly even shoes. For this reason it's best to buy clothing that can expand with you. And I'm not just talking about gear with room for your belly to breathe. I bought a beautiful silk blouse for a special event when I was six months pregnant. It had an empire waist and a loose and flowing midsection so I figured it'd fit well into the third trimester and be a stylish savior after the baby was born. Unfortunately, I didn't take into account that my boobs and upper arms would do their best to keep up with my bump. Two months later, the only part of the blouse that fit was the neck. It never came off of the hanger again.

If practicality is part of your shopping itinerary, stick with stretchy stuff.

Good bras are great investments.

When I first started expanding, I resisted spending money on new clothes, rationalizing that it was a waste since I would only need them for a short time. But before I knew it, my "scoops of flesh" (as they were so adorably deemed in the movie classic "The Sure Thing") were more like buckets of bosom, spilling over the sides of my bras and heading south at flash-flood speed. Feeling thrifty, I stopped by a lingerie outlet at 20 weeks, discovered I'd gone from a perky B to a dripping D, and snatched up a cheap full-figure bra, which I only wore twice because it was uncomfortable. Two weeks later, I dragged my Ds to A Pea in the Pod where I was properly and professionally fitted for two full blown—and very comfy and expensive—hooter harnesses. One was fantastic, sturdy, with straps as wide as suspenders, and only mildly offensive on the eyes. The other, a Spanx bra, was a total waste of money. It looked chic and felt like a silky and uplifting second skin at first, but within two weeks it stretched out so that my triple-scoops could do nothing other than go with gravity.

Alas, with one good bra in hand I still wasn't out of the woods. I had to buy bras on two additional occasions—at 30 weeks and 36 weeks. The first was from a department store where I was again fitted by a pro. The second and final purchase (of a DD) was from a maternity boutique where I was wisely pointed toward a nursing bra rather than a basic model since I was planning to nurse and would soon need a boob bolster with easy nipple access. It was good advice; that bra collection lasted until today. (My breasts bucked convention and decided to stay a little bigger rather than get smaller than their pre-pregnancy size.) It wasn't cheap, but out of all the purchases I made, really comfortable and high-quality bras were the best money spent.

Maternity clothes age in dog years.

It's not quality that makes these full-figured fashions look a decade old after 10 months of wear. It's the frequency in which they are worn and washed. Your maternity selection is probably much smaller than your everyday wardrobe, so you're likely to wear and wash the same items more regularly. Other than buying a closet full of choices, your best defense against premature aging is hand washing, machine washing using the delicate cycle, or dry cleaning your maternity clothes.

Your underwear will suffer.

If you wear G-strings or thongs you may not need to buy larger underwear during your pregnancy because they are likely to fit you even at your fullest. (Although if you develop hemorrhoids, the pain will inspire you to forget about flossing.) But you should put away your fancy pants if you want to wear them after pregnancy, when you can actually look down and admire them again. Otherwise, make a plan to treat yourself to all new undies after the birth. Why? Because no clothing bears the brunt of your percolating pregnant body more than your intimates—unless you regularly wear panty liners (which is a great idea by the way, since pregnancy leakage is potent enough to destroy even the sturdiest stretch cotton).

"Don't try to hide your shape. You'll end up looking like a tent with a head."

Stash your loveliest lingerie away in your deepest drawers and either use your everyday undies or buy a bunch just for the next nine months.

Shopping is depressing.

If you hated shopping before you got pregnant this won't mean anything to you. But if your idea of a fun Saturday is one spent rummaging the racks for new fabulous outfits, brace yourself. There is no bigger bummer than pining over pants that you can't pull up past the knee or blouses that practically burst at the seams just by your looking at them.

Even trips to maternity stores sucked for me. I was very comfortable trouncing my pregnant figure around out in the world, but while twirling in front of the dressing-room mirror it was impossible not to fall prey to my usual self-criticism. Looking through my pre-pregnancy eyes, I saw a distorted funhouse reflection of myself rather than a miracle in the making. (Don't get me wrong. It wasn't the bump that put me off. It was the expansion of everything around it.) Plus much of the comfy clothing that actually fit me was so far from my personal style that I may as well have run off and joined the circus.

If you're prone to self-deprecation, make it easy on yourself by sticking to stores that have clothing that will fit you. Then cast kind glances at yourself in the dressing-room mirror, don't look too hard at yourself until you're dressed, or, when all else fails, head straight to baby stores where you can delight over tiny booties and completely impractical yet irresistibly fabulous newborn fashions.

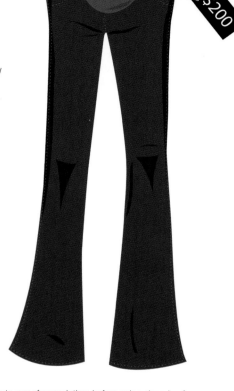

Shopping while desperate

is dangerous. Trust me on this. If you wait until you can't fit into any of your clothes before going shopping for maternity garb, by the time you make your way to a boutique you will spend more than you want to, buy things you might have otherwise passed up, and leave feeling horrible instead of fabulous. Just like grocery shopping while hungry, desperation dressing is never a good idea. If you have the time, browse physical and online shops before you actually need to buy anything. Then, when the time comes, you'll know your options and purchase with style and practicality in mind.

A little makeup and hair

styling goes a long way. If you've ever seen candid photos of celebrities without makeup and hairstyling you know that a little primping can make the difference between a mess and a masterpiece. If you're feeling hopeless, add a little cosmetic fabulousness to your face and style your hair. It should perk you right up.

"Stick to shopping at stores that have clothing that will fit you."

You will never want to see your maternity clothes again

the minute you have your baby. It doesn't matter whether you spent a few dollars or a small fortune on maternity fashions. You will still be way over your wardrobe the second that tot arrives, which is unfortunate since you are likely to have to continue wearing them for several months before you can even think about trying on your old clothes.

FASHION BASICS

There is no right way to work the pregnant look. But there are some basic tips that will help you, whether your idea of dressing up includes a shirt and shoes or a full-blown ball gown.

Put your "regular" clothes into storage.

If you thought you had a closet full of clothes and nothing to wear before you were pregnant, wait until you pop. The minute you can't comfortably fit into your everyday garb, your closet becomes a museum showcasing the old you, which does you no good as you try to decide what to squeeze into today. Besides, browsing through stuff you can't wear is depressing even if you think your new body is the best thing since disposable diapers. And, as already mentioned, forcing yourself into your favorite sweater will stretch it out forever—something you will regret the minute the baby weight falls off.

Consider rearranging your closet so that the wearable stuff is within sight and reach. Tuck away the things you can't wear or want to preserve. It'll alleviate some of the anxiety around getting dressed and make it easier to browse your options.

Don't buy clothes before you fit into them.

Many maternity stores have a fake pregnant tummy that you can strap on while trying on clothes to get an idea of how they'll fit when you're further along. Don't believe the belly hype—unless it comes as a full-on fat suit. It might not be just your midsection that grows, but also the thighs, boobs, upper arms, back flesh, and everything else that matters when you're wiggling into an outfit. Yes, a good sale can inspire a girl to rationalize all kinds of craziness. But if you invest in sizes well beyond your current status, you might end up with a pregnancy wardrobe that's as useful as that favorite old pair of pants in the back of the closet that are waiting for you to return to your high school weight.

Invest in a few great basic pieces.

If you can justify splurging on a fabulous maternity wardrobe, rock on, sister. But most of us have to make do on a budget and the best way to do that is to invest in essentials, embellish with one-size-fits-all accessories (see below for more on those), and finagle a few glam pieces by borrowing or bargain-hunting (more on that later).

"Basic" means many things to many people. To me it translates to clothing that is comfortable, practical for everyday wear, versatile, flattering, good for mixing and matching, and neutral enough that they won't stand out as the exact things you wore yesterday when paired with different accessories.

As I mentioned before, my basics wardrobe included one pair of maternity jeans, a pair of stretchy black pants, several T-shirts (white, black, charcoal, and one fun bright orange number), a few tank tops, a black dress, and black empire-waist blouse, and a roomy cashmere hoody. (I had a hand-me-down white blouse, too, but I never wore it because I was so heavy up top, the sheer expanse of the fabric reminded me of a catamaran setting sail.)

The Rubber Band Trick

The rubber-band pants trick is an old one, but it works when you're just past the point of zipping up your trousers but not large enough to get into maternity gear. To keep wearing your pants a little longer, loop a rubber band through the buttonhole of your pants and then wrap it around the button. You'll need to wear a shirt that covers your unzipped pants, of course, but if you want a few more weeks in your everyday jeans and your hips and thighs are cooperating, this is a good cheap fix.

Buy clothes in complementary colors.

With a limited wardrobe, you need to do a lot of mixing, matching, and reinterpreting so leave the vibrant flair to the accessories and keep your fashions neutral and flexible.

Get one or two special items

that make you feel fabulous. Whether you treat yourself to a gorgeous blouse or score a few exceptional hand-me-downs or resale store finds, it's essential to have one or two pieces that you can throw on when you're going out on the town. It will make the difference between feeling dumpy and dashing. If you need ideas on where to splurge, check out all of your shopping options in Chapter 13.

Cotton underwear is the best.

Whether you're buying new pregnancy panties or wearing what you have on hand, intrinsically breathable cotton is key for yoo-hoo comfort and itch relief. If you're investing, get lots of inexpensive durable pairs that can handle heavy wear and washing and that you won't mind tossing after the fact.

Accessories are your BFFs (best friends forever).

Some good news on the fashion front: Generally speaking, accessories will never betray you. When all else fails, you can—and should—rely on basic outfits and work wonders with bracelets, necklaces, scarves, earrings, hair accessories, handbags, hats, and anything else that can divert you from fashion doldrums and put some sass in your pregnant step. More than one Mommy Menagerie member bought fun new rings to wear when their everyday bands became too

The Mommy Menagerie
On...Ring In The Pregnancy

99 members of the Mommy Menagerie answered the question, "What month did you take off your rings?" For me it was in the eighth month. Read for details on if and when their fingers got too pudgy to partake.

Month	Number of Mommies	Month	Number of Mommies
1	0	6	10
2	2	7	8
3	2	8	11
4	4	9	3
5	9	Never	50

tight, and I was known to tie a colorful ribbon beneath my boobs to create an empire waist look on a snug-fitting basic black dress. Get creative and you can conceptualize a variety of looks without changing your shirt and slacks.

Certain cuts flatter the pregnant figure better

than others. At some point pregnant women may take on a little of the Humpty Dumpty look (impossibly compact maternity models aside). By paying attention to the following tips, you can be a good egg without looking like one.

As one wise mommy pointed out: "**V-necks** create a shape that diverts from your usual pear." I found this to be especially true for pregnant women with huge racks. Show supersized cleavage and most people won't notice anything beneath your bust—or above it!

Clingy T-shirts are attractive, especially if they hug not only your top half but also your belly. Extra breathing room just makes you look larger all the way around.

I was also a fan of the **flowing skirt**, which hung comfortably beneath my belly and hid my thickened thighs—a style that was far less offensive than my pregnancy tracksuit, which actually tied mid-tummy and looked like an egg cup with pant legs.

Low-waist pants are a godsend for tummy girth. I wore my superstretchy everyday jeans until I had seven months and more than 30 additional pounds under my low-waist belt.

Remove the Piercings
If you've got a bellybutton ring, most sources recommend you remove it. It is likely to become irritating, bumping on things as you start to go through life belly-first. Also, if you happen to have a nipple ring and plan to breastfeed, you're all good so long as you remove the piercing beforehand. Word on the street and in the doctor's office is that piercings do not adversely affect the ability to breastfeed.

Shirts and dresses with **empire waists** (waistlines that begin just below the bust) can be especially flattering—unless your boobs are big enough to dwarf your stomach.

Special maternity gear

can be very beneficial. Beyond basic fashions, there are a number of garments designed to make pregnant life easier. You may not need or want any of these items, but if you want to keep wearing your regular pants after you can no longer button them, if you suffer from back problems, or have grown tired of digging deep into your crotch to pull up your so-called, support-top panty hose, read on.

A pregnancy bra: If you've got or are getting large jugs, I can't stress enough how relieving a well-made pregnancy bra can be.

The Bella Band: More than one Mommy Menagerie member turned to this popular elastic belt, which helps hold up your pants during that in-between stage when you're too big to zip your regular slacks and not quite ready for maternity rags. You'll need a long shirt to cover it up—and the band can't do a darned thing if your thighs are also too wide to fit into your pants.

Maternity hose: Built to accommodate your grandeur and feel comfy all day, specialty hose is far more practical than a larger regular size since the top of basic hose will inch down your tummy and uncomfortably bunch around your already overwhelmed crotch.

Nursing tank tops: If you are well into your pregnancy, plan to breastfeed, need tank tops or shirts, and want to save money, skip pregnancy stuff and buy nursing tops. With subtle snaps that allow you to pull out a boob on command, they come in cute styles and will save you from doubling up on duds. For sources on where to fish for these fascinating finds, see Chapter 13.

Pregnancy girdle: It ain't sexy, but a good, sturdy pregnancy girdle can give support and comfort and make you look lovelier in your clothes. There are a number of styles with various levels of back support and benefit, so be sure to get fitted by someone knowledgeable. A favorite of at least one Mommy Menagerie member was SPANX Maternity, which she claims, "Sucked in everything in the butt and thigh area." Who couldn't use a little of that?

BEAUTY BASICS

There were definitely times when my pregnancy "glow" dimmed and I couldn't remember what it was like to look or feel pretty. During these moments I found it best to focus on one tiny feature that recalled the old me, specifically my eyes, fingernails, toenails, and hair (though my tresses were infinitely more thick and radiant while in waiting).

In Chapter 7, I discuss the indulgence factor of beauty treatments. But for the fashionably challenged, a trip to the cosmetic counter, face and body products boutique, manicurist, or hair salon does a lot more than make you feel pampered. It can genuinely make you feel fresh and fabulous again—at least for a little while.

The Mommy Menagerie On …Must-Buy Clothing

105 mommies divulged their absolute must-buy maternity gear. Ranked for your reading pleasure, here are the top five essentials you might consider throwing into your shopping cart.

1. Jeans
28% of mommies considered a dose of denim to be critical.

2. Black Pants
17% of women went for these versatile numbers, which work for day or night, dressing up or dressing down.

3. Maternity or **Nursing Bra**
14% of the vote supported a good bra choice.

4. A Dress, Stylish Blouse, Bella Band, Underwear, and **T-Shirts**
All of the above received 5% of the vote.

5. Pajamas, Sweat Pants, Yoga Pants, and **Tank Tops/Camis**
4% of mommies migrated toward each of these comfy-cute items.

The Mommy Menagerie On ...Fashion Tips

I asked 111 mommies for their best advice on how to stay comfortably chic.
Here are some highlights.

*"Buy sexy underwear. You don't have to buy prego
panties."*

> *"Invest in one pair of really good maternity jeans."*

"Accentuate the positive—your boobs."

> *"Wear maternity tank tops under unbuttoned pre-maternity,
> button-down shirts for a good look."*

*"Black form-fitting tops make you look put together
and can go from day to night."*

> *"A black turtleneck sweater goes with anything or by itself."*

*"Buy one pair of pants that are comfortable and don't
look terrible. I think that's the thing to spend the money
on. After that, it's all just window dressing."*

> *"Stay in the pants that go below your belly as long as pos-
> sible, because when you have to switch to the pants that
> are up above your belly button, you hit an all new fashion
> low. And when you are at that point, you will discover the
> joy and comfort of overalls."*

*"Focus on hair and make-up and on a simple complete
outfit. Accessorizing is key to finishing an outfit."*

"Look around for styles similar to what you wore before you got pregnant. You'll feel more comfortable in the style you've already carved out for yourself, and everyone will see you as chic if you're confident about your style."

"Skirts are a better bet than pants, because you don't want to constantly deal with hitching your pants up. They will creep down, no matter what."

"Weather permitting, wear skirts with boots and pair them with some really funky tights. That was my look and it totally worked for me. I got a lot of compliments and it was clear this wasn't your mama's pregnancy."

"Remember that you will be a hotter person, so avoid long sleeves or warm fabrics."

"Do NOT hold out for a minute! Just get right into those wonderfully comfortable maternity clothes. There are so many cute, fun, fashionable choices, whether you want to hide your belly or show it off. I loved to show it off with fun shirts."

"If you're a hot prego, call local maternity stores and ask if they need a model. You can often get clothes in trade for photos."

"Check the men's section in the thrift store; there are a some fun and roomy clothes to be found."

"Buy extra big clothes that are non-pregnancy until you have to wear the silly stuff."

I got pregnant at a time when a baby "bump" was all the rage in Hollywood and media was, and probably still is, touting pregnancy as sexy. Plenty of magazines showcased women who were living embodiments of just how hot an expecting woman can look—albeit with hair and makeup artists, great lighting, professionally styled ensembles, and most likely some good airbrushing. Out in the world with my freshly pregnant perspective, I also regularly spotted plenty of women who appeared to sashay through the process with style and grace.

I entered my three trimesters excited to rock the pregnant look—and still felt fabulous after I began really packing on the pounds and realized that, due to my short stocky stature and new double-watermelon chest, I was destined to look more Blue Meanie in the Beatles "Yellow Submarine" than a prego Brooke Shields in "The Blue Lagoon." As trimesters wore on, I had plenty of opportunity to indulge in self-loathing—my horrible wardrobe, boobs that had gone the way of cow udders, and a husband who regularly rejected doing the horizontal tango being just three examples. Still, I kept a positive, confident perspective up until very close to the end, when I was just too darned big and uncomfortable to feel anything but over it.

But my secret for self-esteem success had nothing to do with feeling or looking sexy. I nurtured my confidence in a far more internal way—by adopting a perspective that allowed me to cast a completely new and appreciative eye on everything about me: Pregnancy is a powerful, miraculous, and important job with a higher purpose.

This point of view allowed me to appreciate my body for its wondrous abilities, feel empowered and happy, and accept that part of doing a great job may very well include feeling like Willy Wonka's Violet Beaurigard minus the blueberry hue.

Looking in the mirror, I didn't think of myself as my pre-pregnant self, but as a woman making a baby from scratch. And from that perspective, I could only see myself with pride, amazement, a sense of humor, and affection for the cute, roly-poly novelty I had become. As far as I was concerned, I was a VIP who happened to be going to the party *wearing* her plus one rather than arriving on his or her arm. On the rare occasion that my Zen mindset failed me, an eyebrow wax, pedicure, or dash of retail therapy always worked wonders.

HEALTHY WAYS TO SIZE YOURSELF UP

Losing your self-esteem is not a pregnancy prerequisite. In fact, you may feel more fabulous and purposeful than you ever have before. I, for one, definitely wish that for you and hope that you have no reason to read this chapter. But if you ever find yourself looking through the judgmental, self-critical, weight-obsessed mirror that most of us regularly reflect on, you might enjoy a few tips on how to healthily approach and embrace your royally round body. You'll find 'em here, along with insight and empathy from the Mommy Menagerie.

Make peace with the idea of weight gain.

I know this may be easier said than done, but the fact of the matter is that if you are going to do pregnancy right, you should and will gain a good amount of weight. You may be one of those women whose only sign of pregnancy is the basketball-shape under their shirt or you may wear your status from top to toe. Regardless, this is the one time in your life that you can actually get excited when you tip the scale, so revel in it. That said, it's still a good idea to tuck your scale away for the time being—and perhaps even look away when you're weighed at the doctor's office if you're

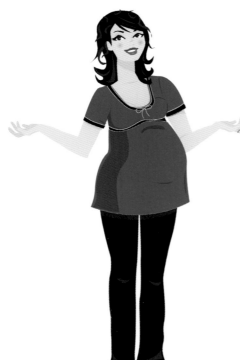

prone to poundage-induced panic. There's no easier way to bum a pregnancy high than to continually obsess on how many ounces you've gained since this morning.

Don't get down on yourself

if your weight gain isn't following the pregnancy chart norms. There are valid reasons why it's not a great idea to gain tons more weight than is recommended (one example is recent studies that connect excessive pregnancy weight to a heightened risk of breast cancer). However, if your path is taking a heavier tack, there's no sense in continually cursing yourself for it. Knowing that I was 10 weeks ahead of the recommended weight-gain schedule within the first three months didn't help me any—or alter my eating, unfortunately. It just made me stop reading books and articles that made me feel bad about myself. I relied on my doctor to tell me if I needed to cut back on the chicken enchiladas—and every time I asked her if I was "overweight," she reassured me that I was doing just fine.

The Mommy Menagerie On ...Did you feel sexy?

On page 166, I list the percentages of mommies who felt stunning, stunted, or otherwise during their nine-month ordeal. But here you'll find a few of my favorite explanations on what it was like to live large.

"Sometimes I felt beautiful, but in a powerful way. . . . can't explain it. I think I felt the most comfortable with my body in my entire life."

"I felt more comfortable in clothes because I wasn't worried about sucking my stomach in for once."

"When I started showing I didn't feel comfortable with the way I looked. I thought that I looked fat and disgusting. As soon as I started getting bigger and my belly started to round out I become a lot more confident in myself and enjoyed being pregnant."

"I think that up to about six months or so, I did feel pretty sexy. That's when you just have the nice belly. After that, I felt like a battle ship."

"The first six months I just felt fat. I felt cuter the more I started showing."

"I loved my pregnant body. I have a big butt and wide hips and, for the first time, I felt like my body was perfectly proportioned."

"Up until about month eight I would say yes. It was my first time with real, honest-to-goodness, cleavage."

"Not sexy, but I knew that I looked good. My hair was shiny, my skin glowed. I kept my figure, but just had a big tummy. I have never received as many compliments in my life as I did when I was pregnant."

"The weight gain was hard for me. I have always been thin, so physically that extra weight was hard (my back hurt so bad) and sleeping at night was very difficult. You do what you can, warm compresses, lots of pillows. But, harder still was the emotional toll of weight gain. I have a distorted self-image to begin with (in my head I know I am thin, but I look and see fat). When I was young I flirted with eating disorders. So, I had to keep myself in check, remember who this weight gain was really for, and what a good thing that was. Also, my husband was incredibly supportive, I had to make sure to keep him in the loop about how I was feeling, so that he could help keep me positive."

"My rear end, hips, and thighs got much bigger and rubbed together. There was nothing I could do but not look down."

"It was hard adjusting to the changing my body was doing. Now when I look back at pictures I say, 'Wow, I looked great pregnant.'"

"I was less body-conscious, which is key for feeling sexy."

Get a fresh perspective.

We are judgmental beings—especially when it comes to ourselves—and I'll bet that despite your fears of what people might think about you, no one is as critical of you as you. In other words, you are your harshest critic. If you find yourself being overly judgmental about the new you, try to remember what you thought when you saw pregnant women before you were in waiting. Was it the sight of their blooming backsides, tragic fashion, or blotchy pregnancy masks that made the greatest impressions? Probably not. More likely you viewed these women with admiration or sympathy—and that's if you noticed them at all, since as I've said previously, most of us are too busy focusing on ourselves to linger too long on others. If you did sum them up, I'll bet you looked at the whole pregnant picture and not just the superficial stuff.

If you're feeling down about the shape of things, remember that people tend to look at pregnant women in a kind and understanding light—especially if the person looking at you is a mother. When we mommies catch a glimpse of a pregnant woman, we instinctually see all the beauty and magic within you because we've been there, know the indescribable joy of what comes next, and are crazy excited for you.

The Mommy Menagerie On ...Did you feel sexy during pregnancy?

Out of the 109 women who answered the question above, some felt sizzling hot, some definitely not. And some even felt dumpy one pregnancy and deliciously sexy the next. Where do you land on the hot mamma scale?

37% answered "No" or "Are you kidding?"

27% said pregnancy did impart sex appeal.

18% sometimes felt the heat.

9% experienced long stints of sexiness after the first trimester or which waned by the third.

4% felt "pretty," "cute," and "beautiful" were more apt descriptors.

3% occasionally felt sexy.

2% experienced no noticeable change.

Weight Gain in Percentages

When I was pregnant I didn't find the recommended weight gain charts helpful since they listed gaining goals rather than realities. So when I conducted the Mommy Menagerie polls, I asked each woman to list how many pounds she actually gained. But I was also interested in results that evened the pre-pregnancy-weight playing field, so I asked each mommy to divide the number of pounds she gained into her pre-pregnancy weight to discover what percentage of her original body weight she gained as well. Where do you weigh in? Read on!

Pounds Gained	% of Pregnancies
0-15 pounds:	<1%
16-20 pounds:	9%
21-25 pounds:	10%
26-30 pounds:	24%
31-35 pounds:	20%
36-40 pounds:	17%
41-45 pounds:	9%
46-50 pounds:	4%
51-55 pounds:	3%
56-60 pounds:	2%
61-65 pounds:	1%
65+ pounds:	<1%

% Weight Gain	% of Pregnancies
0-15% of pre-pregnancy body weight:	13%
16-20% of pre-pregnancy body weight:	11%
21-25% of pre-pregnancy body weight:	28%
26-30% of pre-pregnancy body weight:	22%
31-35% of pre-pregnancy body weight:	13%
36-40% of pre-pregnancy body weight:	11%
40+% of pre-pregnancy body weight:	2%

Accept the things you cannot change.

Lamenting the fact that my breasts were reaching for my belly button wouldn't have been any more productive than wishing my husband lusted after my new wide load; I'd still have been left hanging in both situations. Better to take nothing personally and rock on with your round self.

If you don't like something

about your pregnant body, don't look at it!

When I was 17 and visited Hawaii, there was a tremendous amount of cat road-kill on the highway. Each day when we barreled down the road headed for surf and sun I'd take hard looks at the sad mangled mounds of fur and become traumatized and heartbroken for half the morning. Finally a friend recommended a ridiculously simple yet smart solution. She said, "The minute you see that distant bump in the road, make a point of not looking at it." From then on I diverted my gaze at the first inkling of a flattened Fluffy. Sure it was a simple act of denial, but I have been forever less tormented because of it.

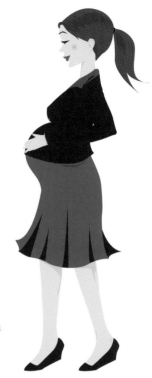

I applied the same notion to my overly bulbous backside when I was about seven months pregnant. Rather than stand in the full-length mirror and rubberneck like a driver passing a car wreck, I decided that the best defense against unpleasant body changes is not to look at them. If you're troubled by any element of your temporary physique, try my friend's tactic and see if in this case ignorance really is bliss for you, too.

Tell your partner to lie.

If your partner doesn't know the requisite answer to the question, "Do I look fat?" or "Does this make me look fat?" now's the time to clue in the jury. In all discussions around weight and beauty, especially when your whole body begins to resemble a sausage, the only answer is, "I've never seen you look more beautiful."

Focus on your baby.

One of the best ways that I became more accepting of my body was to develop an active relationship with my unborn baby. From reading her bedtime stories through feeling her regular bouts with the hiccups (now that was weird!) to playing gentle games of knock-knock, the magical connection reminded me of my purpose and made becoming a human balloon trivial in comparison.

Remember that confidence is sexy.

When I was in high school and completely convinced that I was unlovable and overweight at 114 pounds (sigh), I witnessed something that changed my understanding of beauty forever. One of my most popular—and fit—girlfriends

> *You Are Cute!*
> No matter how funky you think you look now, when you see photos of your pregnant self later you will be surprised at how cute you were.

started seriously plumping up yet she remained as desired and admired by women and men because of one simple thing: she acted like she was hot. She was so comfortable in her body that her attraction was irresistible. From that day forward, I unknowingly following the self-help mantra, "Fake it 'til you make it," and pretended I had self-confidence until it eventually became genuine. Ultimately, I was left with this absolute: Perky boobs and washboard tummies can come and go but lasting beauty is one that radiates from the inside out. Add this philosophy to your emotional wardrobe, wear it regularly, and you will be stunning whether you squeeze into your low-slung jeans or work the tent look.

Buy yourself something that makes you feel pretty.

One of the easiest ways to bring yourself out of the self-esteem dumps is to splurge on something that makes you feel beautiful. It can be as simple as a new lip liner and gloss or as elaborate as a haircut or color, eyebrow wax, mani/pedi, cosmetic-counter makeover, or a fabulous maternity blouse or nightie. Treat yourself as deserving and you will begin to believe it.

The Weight Gain Cheat Sheet

One of the things I yearned for while in waiting was someone to compare myself to, even if it was pointless since all pregnancies are different and there is no "right" way for it to go. Regardless, rather than the annoying weight-gain guidelines, which always made me feel like I was the only woman out there who fell off the optimum weight-gain chart, I'm offering you a slice of real-life pregnancy pounds. So here it is—my gaining schedule ounce for ounce. Feel free to chart yours here, too.

Week Gestation	Erika's Weight	My Details
0	122	_____
8	129	_____
13	129.5	_____
18	138	_____
22	143	_____
26	150	_____
30	153	_____
31	157	_____
32	154.5	_____
34	157	_____
36	159	_____
37	161	_____
38	162	_____
39	162	_____
40	163	_____

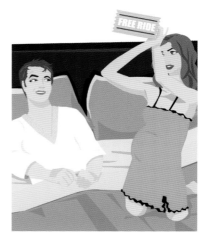

If you ask me what my number-one pregnancy craving was, the answer would have to be sex. I wanted it so much and so often that had I been married to an 18-year-old in his sexual prime, he probably still would have had to regularly pop Viagra to keep up with my libido. Ironically, once I was showing, my usually lascivious husband was about as interested in sex as he was in cleaning the cat box.

Luckily I can usually stop myself from making other people's issues my own, so rather than harboring resentment toward Colie, feeling unattractive, or simply giving up and going without, I accepted my husband's feelings (or rather lack of them), gossiped with girlfriends who had similar dilemmas, and made do.

Every now and then, when times got really tough, I strategically encouraged Colie to relax and watch a steamy movie with me—something I never did otherwise. Sure enough, a few minutes into the on-screen shenanigans the opportunity would arise. Turns out many of my girlfriends found this tactic to be very effective as well.

Closer to my due date, I appealed for sympathy sex once or twice, reasoning that a good roll in the hay might induce labor. (It didn't, but my husband humored me, bless his heart.)

But mostly, I just let it alone. Heaven knows pressure and obligation sex is a surefire way to smolder even the strongest bedroom flames. Instead I found the humor in it all—and reminded myself that sometime in the future my body and our bedroom would be popular frolicking grounds once again. Good thing I didn't know exactly how far in the future it would be. I hope it's different for you but, in our household, the exhaustion of sleepless early months and a baby in the bedroom made regular nights of passion about as likely as winning the lottery without buying a ticket.

ROMANCING WHILE ROUND-BELLIED

A pregnant sex life can be sensational, stifled, or depressing, depending on the circumstances, parties involved, emotions and communication skills at hand, and desire or lack thereof.

Fortunately, there's more than one way to keep the romance alive. You'll find ways to do that here, along with important facts, preferred positions, and everything else you may not want to ask Mom.

Given that you're reading this book you obviously know how to have sex. But you may not be as well versed in the particulars of pregnancy sex. If you're the least bit curious—and who isn't? It's sex after all!—read on for things you might want to know before you stumble upon them beneath the sheets.

Sex will not be the same

as it was before. Whether you consider lovemaking a task you check off your honey-do list or rank it right up there with chocolate, free money, and fabulous shoes, sex is bound to be different now. You can chalk up some of the change to your body's increased blood volume which, when aroused, can incite swelling that hasn't been seen since Marsha Brady's nose had that fateful collision with a football. Only it'll be your sexually stimulated vagina that looks like it has been supersized (and it may feel tighter upon entry, too). You can also point to haywire hormones, which early on can make you as dry as the desert (use lubrication!), and later as free flowing as a mountain stream. And let's not forget that it isn't long before a certain third wheel is clearly in bed with you, and possibly even kicking along as you bump and grind. (If you or your partner finds this unnerving, it helps to remember that your baby hasn't the foggiest idea what you're doing, but does piggyback on your feelings, and thus reap the benefits of your relaxed, feel-good vibes.) Best of all, orgasms tend to intensify, become multi-orgasmic, or both—and what's not to like about that?

High-Risk Warning

If you are considered high-risk for preterm labor, forgo intercourse, nipple stimulation, and any type of orgasm until you check with your practitioner. While these playful activities are safe for the everyday pregnant woman, they could prematurely get the ball rolling for the at-risk mommy-to-be.

Your desire for sex may change.

Some women become virtual sex machines, while others suddenly consider doing the laundry more exciting. It's also entirely possible to roller coaster between these diametric stances, depending on the trimester, your self-image, and myriad other factors that regularly incite a woman to feel frisky or frigid.

Unfortunately, though partners may not be able to relate to the pregnant plight, they are subject to it, so communicating your ups and downs and emphasizing that it's a hormonal thing is very helpful.

Whatever the case, you should definitely embrace your sexual stance and remember that like so many other elements of your pregnancy—including pregnancy itself—the situation is temporary. So have fun with your newfound passion for abstinence or excess. Soon you'll have an entirely new situation that's equally likely to affect your sex life in unexpected ways.

Your partner's desire

for sex may change. Your partner may not have the hormone excuse, but there are plenty of factors that can affect your lover's libido, from parenting fears to seeing you more as a holy vessel than a naughty minx, to difficulty adjusting to being the slighter of the two in the lovemaking lair. Some partners are perfectly willing to discuss such matters, while others may not be, and that's not necessarily a bad thing. Some things are better left unsaid to the pregnant woman, especially if it has anything to do with a limp sexual libido as a result of pregnancy weight. In such cases, I'd personally rather hear a polite lie than press for a painfully honest answer.

Orgasmic Tremors
If you want to feel something way cool, when you have an orgasm well into your pregnancy immediately put your hand on your tummy. You will feel your entire belly (actually your uterus) contract and getting very firm to the touch. Don't worry, it's temporary and normal.

If you're not feeling the love and are struggling with it, do your best to accept the things you cannot change, know that the situation is temporary, and consider satisfying yourself.

Orgasms are better than ever.

Whether self-induced or gifted, orgasms are safe and fabulous for the pregnant woman, so long as she does not have a high-risk of preterm labor, in which case they could potentially induce labor. Orgasms are also now more orgasmic, literally, and should by all means be experienced and enjoyed as much as desired. The only exception is the very rare circumstance that they inspire continual uterine contractions. In that case, you should call your practitioner immediately.

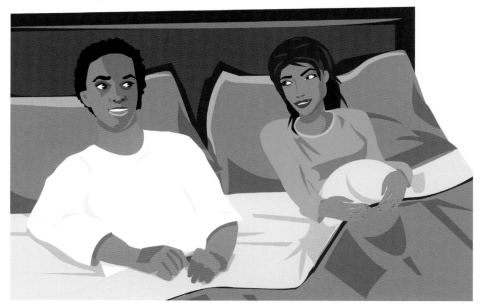

Your body is your best sexual barometer.

As with all aspects of pregnancy, your body will tell you what it wants, likes, and needs. So like everything else, when it comes to sex, follow your instincts and your body's reactions. The best sexual position for you is the one that feels good. If something doesn't feel good, causes cramping, or is just plain uncomfortable, don't do it. That includes satisfying your partner, by the way. If you're not into it, blame it on the hormones and let him fend for himself.

Sex talk is important.

You may not need to discuss birth control until just before your due date, but there are all kinds of fun sexual topics that demand attention during your nine-month adventure. Some issues are sensitive and require creative solutions or at least acknowledgement and reassurance—like an unrequited lack or excess of sexual libido. Others are more about finesse, such as sharing things you don't want to do because they hurt, or ways to make sex more comfortable given your new girth.

> "Orgasms are also now more orgasmic, literally, and should be enjoyed as much as desired."

If you and your partner are well versed in bedroom banter, you're likely to enjoy sharing the peaks and valleys that come with pregnancy and sexual intimacy. But if talking openly isn't usually your thing, you might want to step outside of your comfort zone. It's especially important to say what works and doesn't work for your body now because even if your partner knew those details yesterday, they are likely to change tomorrow— and possibly forever. (One of my previous foreplay favorites—nipple stimulation—became a total turn off the minute I got pregnant and I still can't stand it to this day. Mommy friends say the same is true for them.)

Besides, sexual intimacy isn't solely achieved through the act of lovemaking. It's also about you and your partner sharing feelings, fears, and desires—and being loving, understanding, respectful, and resourceful when you find yourselves on opposite sides of the bed. And trust me, with a baby-size bulge and a body pillow between you, that's likely to happen on more than one occasion.

By the way, your newly open channels of communication will remain in your relational repertoire, provided you use them regularly.

KEEP ROMANCE ALIVE

There are many reasons to consider alternatives to sex during pregnancy, foremost of which are a disinterested partner and a high-risk pregnancy. But neither of those things means you can't have a satisfying sex life. Whether you want some simulated whoopee with the one you love or plan to go it alone, here are some thoughts to ponder.

The Mommy Menagerie On ...The Top Five Power Positions

Need bedroom inspiration or just want to compare notes? 102 members of the Mommy Menagerie offer a proverbial peek under the covers on the most comfortable ways to do the pregnant wild thing.

1. Doggie Style
Considering that taking it from behind while on all fours ranked number one with a whopping 32% of the vote, this pose, which is especially preferred late in the game, deserves a more dignified name—perhaps "preggie style."

2. Spooning
Whether it was front-to-front or front-to-back, legs together or akimbo, this cuddly side-lying standard was stiff competition for the top position with a 31% approval rating.

3. On Top
Also described by one Menagerie member as "Cowgirl," this comfy woman-on-top, ride 'em pose lassoed 23% of the vote.

4. Missionary
Yup! 13% of the Menagerie managed to lie on their backs with the partner on top well into waiting, although some eased into other satisfying stances once their bellies really bulged.

5. None
For a solid 7% of the Menagerie there was no such thing as the best position. Explanations included: "Had to stop having traditional sex around 16 weeks due to twin pregnancy," "None in particular when you are petrified of squashing baby," and another idea altogether of the perfect position, "Passed out alone on the bed."

Intimacy doesn't have to include sex.

If you can think back to childhood crushes, you might recall that some of the hottest romantic interludes were the least sexual. With the right person, the touch of a hand, stroke of the hair, nibble on the neck, or even thoughtful gaze can make the heart skip a beat. I'll be the first one to tell you that the drudgery of everyday life tends to stop sweaty-palmed moments from regularly occurring at my house. But every now and then when Colie and I create enough mental space to just relax and enjoy each other, magic has been known to happen.

Should you want to sprinkle a little pixie dust on a celibate love life, instigate the opportunity to enjoy a simple shared pleasure, be it dinner in bed, a date at the ball game, a night of dancing (this really does it for us), or a casual walk—provided your partner is willing and interested.

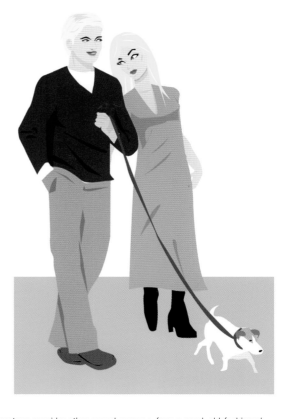

You can have great sex without penetration.

If the actual act of intercourse is frightening, unappealing, or doesn't feel right to you or your partner, consider other sexual avenues, from a good, old-fashioned make-out session to mutual masturbation (a favorite among many men) to your favorite forms of foreplay. A kink in your regular sex routine can result in surprisingly fun adventures if you and your partner are game and have a little creativity.

You can have great sex

without a partner. If you haven't already, it's never too late to discover (and rediscover) the joys of self-pleasure. Plainly put, for the sexually insatiable pregnant woman, one in the hand is virtually better than two in the bed. And if you're adventurous enough to buy a vibrator, it may be more satisfying than ice cream, peanut butter and pickles, and chocolate cake all rolled into one. But good old elbow grease does the trick too.

Amorous Labor Inducer

Along with eating spicy foods, having sex is said to be a possible aid in inducing labor when you're full term because when your body is ready to birth, an orgasm can jumpstart the process. And even when it doesn't work, it can be fun to try.

The Mommy Menagerie On ...A Partner's Lust Level

Just how far does the scale slide when it comes to a partner's sex drive? Check out the following answers to the question, "If you had one, did your partner want to have sex during pregnancy?" and see for yourself.

"Every second of the day."

"Yes, just as much as before. I'm always amazed at how sexy he finds me while I'm pregnant."

"Yep, that was the hardest part—pardon the pun."

"Remarkably, we probably had more sex than we did before I got pregnant."

"Yes. He thought pregnancy made me even more 'sexy' in that mother earth kinda way. I did not feel particularly sexy with such drastic changes going on in my outward appearance, but he always complimented me and tried to make me see the beauty in the change."

"Yes, until the last month or so. Once the baby's head was positioned downwards (or dropped), he felt 'weird' about having intercourse. I suspect it was more the fact that I could have suffocated him under my weight, but I choose to believe what he says."

"He is too sweet to initiate, so I do, even though my libido is low. I feel so bad for the poor guy."

"Yes! However, he was gone on business a lot so I had to resort to self-fulfillment. . . . I felt like a teenage boy!"

"No, I kind of knew it was going to be a sexless pregnancy because we were trying for so long, and he would feel
sex was a risk. Of course the doctors also either prohibited
or discouraged sex, especially in the beginning."

"My husband did not show an interest in sex when I was
pregnant. We had sex only four or five times during the
entire term, which was unfortunate. He told me often that
he thought I was so sexy and beautiful and looked so 'hot'
as a pregnant woman, but that definitely did not translate
to sexual desire on his part."

"Before I got pregnant, we were having sex every day
because the fertility specialist said I was ovulating early
sometimes and late other times. I have no beautiful story
to tell my daughter as I believe the night she was conceived, I yelled, 'Just hurry up and finish.' We had both
had it, and I believe it took us a full year to get
our intimacy back. We had sex maybe five times
during the pregnancy."

"He did, but between stress levels, and then as I got
bigger, no matter how much I assured him it was ok, he
was not that comfortable and was unnerved by thinking
he might somehow harm the babe. We even talked to the
OB-GYN, but the idea still stuck."

"Not the second time, because he wanted to avoid a
miscarriage again and didn't want to do anything that he
thought might contribute to that (even though we knew
that was most likely not a factor at all)."

"Not once I started showing."

The Mommy Menagerie On …Whether Pregnancy Increased or Decreased Sexual Desire

Out of the 82 women who divulged the details:

45% wanted more whoopee.

40% had less interest.

8% were neither here nor there.

5% were foiled by elements such as low self-esteem or medical restrictions.

The Mommy Menagerie On …Did your partner want sex?

Looks like most of the Menagerie got lucky a lot more than me while in waiting—or at least had the opportunity. Out of 111 women:

80% said that their partners wanted sex.

7% of partners didn't.

1% answered "sometimes."

12% fell into the "other" category with explanations ranging from moments of discomfort, fear of hurting the baby late in pregnancy, daddy feeling awkward about having sex with a baby between them, and leaving initiation up to the woman.

Sex Cheat Sheet

 Is intercourse safe while pregnant?

As discussed in Chapter 1, getting down is all good from the moment you conceive until you go into labor. According to the medical pros, all positions are safe, so feel free to do it any which way your hedonistic heart desires as long as you have a consenting partner and do not have premature labor problems, a long legacy of miscarriages, or a diagnosed high-risk pregnancy. In any of those cases it's important to chat with your practitioner before hitting the sheets. (Other reasons to resist until you consult a pro are bleeding, placenta previa—an abnormal implantation of the placenta near the internal opening of the uterine cervix—infection, and amniotic fluid leakage.)

 What about oral sex?

I don't know about you, but considering the aromatic goo factory that my nether regions became midway through pregnancy I thought it unkind to even tilt my husband's head toward the south. But maybe your situation is different (lucky girl), or you haven't reached the saturation point so to speak, or you can wash away any worries with a quick swipe of a dampened facecloth. In any case, oral enjoyment is more than okay to give and receive for the entire duration. In fact, it can be a sexual savior for the frisky family that is not comfortable with penetration and pregnancy or has been advised by professionals not to partake. The exception is if you or your partner is HIV positive since it's possible to share the virus through tissue-to-tissue contact.

One curious word of warning from the pros is not to blow air into the vagina because it can create a potentially lethal air bubble in one of your blood vessels. I don't know where this idea came from or who figured it out, since no woman I know considers being ballooned a remotely stimulating notion. (Perhaps it was some naive soul who took the idea of the blowjob literally.) In any case, if this information isn't enough to make you jump out of your skin at the first hint that your partner is about to sneeze while between your legs, I don't know what is.

 Is anal sex kosher?

Given that most participating partners don't openly discuss the details of rear entry it's not surprising that there aren't any conclusive studies on pregnancy and anal sex. However, there is a generally shared bottom line, and it applies to all pregnancy activities: Do what feels good. If something doesn't feel right or becomes uncomfortable, stop immediately, and be careful not to be too aggressive or forceful.

 How about sex toys or other provocative props?

Not all playthings are created equal. Vibrators and other stand-in stimulators are generally accepted with the caveats that depth of penetration should never be aggressive or forced and use should be discontinued if there is any pain or discomfort. However, generally speaking the integration of foreign objects, be it air, liquid, or solids, is a definite no-no and could be fatal to your fetus.

While shopping for my maternity wardrobe was pure torture, prepping my daughter's room was the exact opposite. My unnecessary sense of urgency aside, conceptualizing the palace for my little princess was one of the sweetest elements of pregnancy. It was the time that I really focused on what was to come, pouring all of my dreams of cuddles and lullabies, tiny toe kisses, and toothless grins into my choice of draperies, type of changing table, and style of rocking chair.

The more the room came together the more real the pending arrival of our new family member became. Admittedly, I was one of those mommies who had to have everything in place in advance, although I did overlook the most practical things like a truckload of diapers. (I foolishly started with one measly pack and a few stragglers doled out by the hospital.) Still, for me there was nothing like the magic of a sweetly decorated nursery in waiting. With the curtains hung, the wall graced with block letters spelling my daughter's name, and the planet's cutest and tiniest teal espadrilles dangling from a child-size coat rack on the wall, I couldn't pass the room without catching my breath. The pride and excitement was overwhelming.

We moved when Viva was seven weeks old—and she slept in our room until long after that—so we never actually spent much time in that room other than to change diapers or rock the baby in the wee hours while one of us got some much-needed shuteye in our bedroom. But I have a photo of it—the big white crib, crisp pink and white sheet, bumper bows retied multiple times because they had to look just right, sea foam green walls, thick cream-colored curtains with matching green line drawings of nursery-rhyme characters, and a cluster of pastel stuffed animals perched on the dresser. Each time I pull out that picture my heart and eyes well up. It reminds me of where you are now: standing at the threshold of a new, deeply challenging and rewarding phase of life, excitedly waiting to meet this wondrous person inside of you, and, if you're a first-timer, not yet knowing just how intense it is to love anyone as much as you will love your child. It's a once-in-a-lifetime place to be.

The truth is, you can get by without all of the prep work I did. Heck, I have a friend whose mom kept her in a padded dresser drawer on the bedroom floor for her first several months of life. But if you've got the time and desire, you might as well go to town now. It's been nearly two years since we moved and I still want to paint the walls and hang more artwork, if only I could finish unpacking the Great Wall of Boxes we ditched in the garage when we first arrived. I'm sure it'll happen—after I get through the perpetual pile of laundry, organize my scattered office, and finish my deadlines, which hopefully will be sometime before my child has a baby of her own.

SHOPPING FOR YOU

Whether you want maternity jeans, belly-hugging shirts, or snuggly PJs, this section gives you enough choices to traipse through all three trimesters in comfort and style. But be sure to brush up on each store's return policy before you commit. Most of the online sources listed below accept returns within a specific timeframe ranging from one week to three months, although intimates and sale items tend to be final. A receipt and the attached original tags are usually required and refunds rarely include shipping costs in either direction, which is one more reason to shop with care.

If you want suggestions and guidance before you set off on a shopping spree, see Chapter 10, which is completely dedicated to the style and substance of pregnancy fashion.

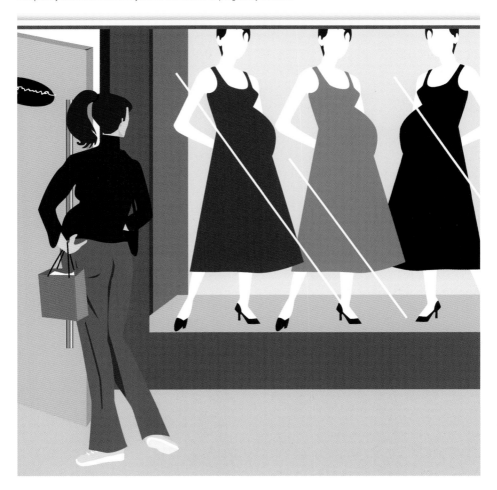

Affordable Options

Craigslist

www.craigslist.com

If you haven't already, you will learn to love this garage sale-like site when it comes time to unload all of your expensive baby contraptions. But you can reap its benefits beforehand if you scour its pages for all things maternity— provided you're cool with wearing nearly new stuff. A recent glance among the gazillion local postings showed a woman in my neighborhood hawking a new $200 pair of designer maternity jeans for $100 or best offer, while a few neighborhoods away I could grab four cute maternity tops for five bucks each.

Ebay

www.ebay.com

There is so much stuff being sold on this website that browsing could be overwhelming. Rather than searching for something generic like "maternity jeans," which garnered 2,579 results when I typed it into their search box, it's better to narrow the options. If searching for jeans, try including your size or desired brand in the search box along with the word "maternity." A search on the words "maternity," "7 For All Mankind jeans," and "size 28" garnered a

The Mommy Menagerie On ...The Best Maternity Stores

107 mommies bellied up with their favorite resources for roundwear. Check out their Top 10 choices.

Store	% of Mommies That Dug It
1. Old Navy	30%
2. The Gap	20%
3. Motherhood	15%
4. Target	10%
5. A Pea In The Pod or Japanese Weekend	9%
6. Local boutiques or Mom's The Word	8%
7. Due Maternity or H&M	7%
8. BabyStyle	6%
9. Second-hand stores	5%
10. Kohl's	3%

total of seven results with prices ranging from $32 to $89 for used denim that usually costs $115 to $175 a pop. Alas, there are no returns, so consider carefully before bidding or buying.

H&M
www.hm.com

As this book goes to press there's no online shopping with this chain known for inexpensive, relatively durable, and impossibly trendy attire. But you can create and dress your own mirror-image model, which I found to be a pretty fun diversion. Still, the Mommy Menagerie tells me that this department store, which regularly recruits famous guest designers (think Stella McCartney and Madonna), sells some great maternity pieces at legendarily low prices. Check the website to find a store near you or see if they've joined the Internet shopping revolution.

JC Penney
www.jcp.com

The selection for big mamma gear is small and not incredibly inspired, but staple pieces like a cute pencil skirt for 20 bucks or empire waist sundress for $30 makes this site, and store, worth a peek.

Kohl's
www.kohls.com

This department store has a limited but attractive selection of basic tops and bottoms by "Oh Baby! By Motherhood" brand. Styles and colors lean toward classic and conservative, which means power mommies may even find a sensible suit among the options. Prices are extremely reasonable and, if you order something you don't want, you can skip paying return postage by bringing the unwanted wear to a retail location.

Motherhood
www.motherhood.com

Site navigation is clunky and some fashions are more mamma mia than hot mamma, but dig deep and you'll find a great selection of staples at extremely good prices. One Mommy Menagerie member stopped here for underwear and basics like a good old black turtleneck. Regardless, with T-shirts topping out at around $20, it's a site worth scouring for even one great find. And with a 30-day return policy, you've got plenty of time to see if a questionable purchase grows on or with you.

Old Navy
www.oldnavy.com

You really can't beat Old Navy's prices or selection. They've got every casual category and size covered, from jeans and cargos to dresses to bathing suits to PJs—all spanning from XS to XXL. Plus there's a perpetual online sale so many items sell for under $10. But discounts

Body Pillow Sources

These cuddly bedroom buddies come in a large array of shapes, sizes, and prices. You can easily comparison shop through an online search, or go straight for sure things. Good sources for inexpensive lounge logs include Target, Amazon.com, Overstock.com, and Bedbathandbeyond.com, while SitInComfort.com sells a vast selection of superposh pillows.

notwithstanding, it's hard to balk at retail prices that top out around $35. Better still, there is a standard $5 shipping and return policy (with a prepaid envelope), so you can return your goods within 90 days without getting off of the couch. Or choose to exchange or waddle into a store near you and the return is free. Of course you get what you pay for, so items may not live to be honored hand-me-downs, but on the bright side, you won't feel so bad chucking them the second you're able to downsize.

Target
www.target.com

Maternity designer Liz Lange is behind Target's broad collection of mommy-to-be wear. Substantially cheaper than her label sold in her namesake boutiques, the pants, tops, dresses, sweater sets, tunics, and hoodies don't push any fashion boundaries, but they are tasteful, classic, and above all, cheap. Free shipping on orders over $50 is an added bonus.

Walmart
www.walmart.com

If the words "dirt cheap" sound good to you, check out your local Walmart or visit their online shop. Last I looked there were some sweet $8 tank tops, $14 capri lounge pants, and $25 Levi maternity jeans showcased alongside dresses and patterned tops that are probably better left on the rack.

Moderately Priced Maternity Gear

Babystyle
www.babystyle.com

This site and its retail locations teeter between bargain prices and splurges. BabyStyle brand items are more affordable and feature T-shirts for under $20 and jeans for around $90. Steeper-priced picks include designer denim that'll set you back close to $200. Fashion is playful but not too funky or trendy, which works just fine for many middle-of-the-road mommies who still want to look smart. While you're in the neighborhood, check out their great kids clothes, toys, accessories, and furniture.

Euphoria Maternity
www.euphoriamaternity.com

A huge selection of T-shirts and dresses are just two appealing reasons to scan this site featuring cute and trendy clothing, most of which is under $100. Browse and you'll find brands such as Japanese Weekend, Lait Maternity, and Childish, as well as good nursing bras by Bravado.

Fit Maternity
www.fitmaternity.com

Refreshingly down to earth, this website featuring real-life mommy models is a great source for tasteful maternity workout clothes at decent prices. Jog by for everything from yoga pants to tummy-friendly tennis garb and you can at least look sporty, even if the extent of your exercise is reaching for the TV remote.

The Gap

www.gap.com

Classic staples are the name of the game at this national chain, which offers garb that runs the size gamut, from 0 to 20. As suggested by the fanfare of the Mommy Menagerie, their diverse and affordable denim is particularly noteworthy. With no panel-, hidden panel-, demi panel-, and roll panel-styles you're likely to find something that fits. Of course other essentials are here, too, from casual skirts to tops to undies to PJs. If you're feeling lazy, shop online and you can return rejects to a local outpost.

Maternity Mall

www.maternitymall.com

Overly complicated navigation makes finding the fashion a bit odious, but this megasite does cover a lot of shopping ground by offering garb from Motherhood, A Pea in the Pod, and Mimi Maternity as well as supercheap stuff like nursing T's for under $17. Alas, if you buy something you don't like you can't take it to a store; online orders must be shipped back.

Mothercare

www.mothercare.com

First the good news: This site has fabulously chic fashions at really good prices. Now the bad: It's U.K. based, which means to understand costs you need to translate British pounds to American dollars (still a great value) and if you want to return anything you'll need to pay for overseas shipping—and get it back to them within 28 days. Still, I would have rocked the Mothercare look had I known about it. Their staples are too stylish and sensibly priced to ignore.

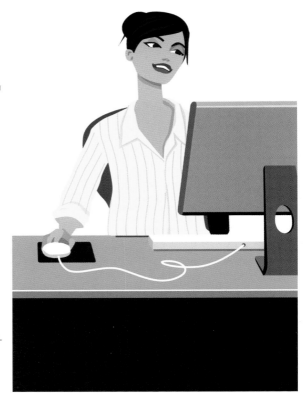

Pricy Picks

2 chix

2chix.com

Perky pick-me-ups in the form of fun, funny T-shirts are the sensation at this website where cute styles come hand-in-hand with clever sayings like "what's kickin'," "haute mama," and "who's your daddy."

A Pea in the Pod

www.apeainthepod.com

A notoriously pricey and hot pick for cute, trendy, good-quality gear, this national chain features virtually all the popular brands—including 7 for All Mankind, Betsey Johnson, Lilly Pulitzer, Juicy Couture, Da Nang, and Cosabella—as well as an astounding array of great tops. Great site organization allows you to search by brand, browse their denim boutique, or cherry-pick through specific types of clothing.

Belly Dance Maternity

www.bellydancematernity.com

Impulse shoppers beware! This site has a dizzying selection of designer options. Shop by brand or clothing type or go straight to sale items by clicking on the red tag in the website's upper right hand corner. But think before you buy. As with most shops, sale items are non-refundable.

Childish

www.childish.com

Self-described as hip, sexy, smart, comfy, sassy, and funky, this company featuring maternity wear—and kid's clothes—is just that, though I'd add youthful, trendy, and clingy to the list. Don't pass up this place if you're counting pennies; sales make splurging on a playful dress more palatable to the budget-minded, fashion-famished mommy.

> "Be sure to brush up on each store's return policy before you commit to a purchase."

Chira Kruza

www.chirakruza.com

If I had known about the fabulous maternity duds sold here I would definitely have indulged. Sophisticated and more chic than trendy, the dresses, tops, and bottoms are favorites with celebrities-in-waiting. Regular online sales make a splurge doable, while their seven-day return policy means if you buy and don't want something, you'd better shuffle to the post office quickly. If you'd rather shop locally, check their site for stores carrying their stuff.

Due Maternity

www.duematernity.com

A cornucopia of fashionable, classic, and practical finds awaits at this very well-organized site. Single-minded mommies-to-be can easily find exactly the type of top, bottom, dress, or active gear they are interested in by selecting from categories such as "stylish," "basic," "novelty," and "strapless." Also stop here for skincare, diaper bags, and nursing stuff, too, and check their store locator, found at the bottom of the page, if you want to find a shop near you.

Japanese Weekend
www.japaneseweekend.com

The sheer volume of trendy tops should inspire you to visit this site, especially since there seems to always be some on sale. But there's more, including light pajama sets, pants, and cute coats and sweaters.

The Mommy Menagerie's
Top Five Maternity Jeans Brands

108 mommies offered insight into the brand of maternity jeans that they bought. Want to know what topped the charts? While 7% vetoed jeans altogether and 10% went for hand-me-downs, the other 83% did their pregnancy in purchased denim. Try the following labels on for size.

1. The Gap
25% of mommies preferred the classic cuts from this national retailer.

2. Old Navy
13% went for the wonderfully inexpensive options sold at this clothier.

3. 7 for All Mankind
This designer style reigned supreme with 8% of the vote.

4. Japanese Weekend or **Motherhood Maternity**
It was a two-way tie for these bump-friendly boutiques, each of which received praise by 7% of mommies.

5. Mimi Maternity or **Citizens of Humanity**
The maternity boutique and designer brand face off for a two-way tie with 2% of the vote each.

Liz Lange

www.lizlange.com

The inspiration behind designer Liz Lange's Target line, the maternity wear here is the high-end real deal, with seasonally changing styles that are all-around classic, great-looking, and well-made. They're also far more womanly-chic than girly-cute, and include outstanding outfits for the office and special occasions.

Maternal America

www.maternalamerica.com

This site's glam shots of ridiculously luminous and slender pregnant women are about as good for the self-image as a nice fat pimple on the tip of your nose. But the clothing sure is chic. From urban denim to feminine floral dresses to Pucci-like printed tops, the clothing here is about as stylish as it gets.

Mimi Maternity

www.mimimaternity.com

This chain store's private-label trendy wear comes to the rescue of the fashionable femme looking for virtually everything from maternity wear to wedding dresses to yoga gear. While it's young in look and spirit, there are some sure-fire staples to be found here, too.

Mom's The Word

www.momsthewordmaternity.com

As designer brand central, this California-based shop is where fancy and well-funded mommies can stop for ga-ga friendly garb by trendy sources such as Velvet, Michael Stars, Diane von Furstenburg, and Chaiken.

Veronique Maternity

www.veroniquematernity.com

Here she is: The big mama of expensive, gorgeous designer clothes. If you're on a tight budget, even peeking at the enviable garb here may make your credit card break a sweat. But fortunately, it'll take more than a point and click to blow your wardrobe wad on the stunning French, Italian, and American designs showcased on the site. You can browse the collection online, but you'll have to call the store to purchase.

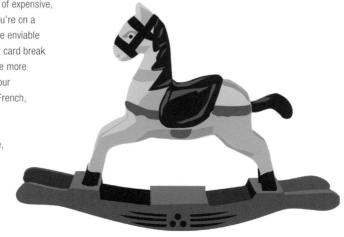

SHOPPING FOR BABY

Buying for Baby is a slippery slope. You head to the store with the specific agenda of finding a changing table pad or nose aspirator, but stumble onto infinite painfully adorable things that you don't need but absolutely have to have. I found this to be especially true of clothing, although when I was five months pregnant I did rationalize buying a ridiculously expensive rocking horse that neighed and made galloping sounds when you pinched its ears; it's been two years and counting since then and Viva's still not old enough to ride it, but boy does it look cute in her room.

Then there are those treacherous layette lists, which dictate everything you should load up on before Baby comes and often include more than you really need. (A layette is just a fancy word for a set of newborn's essential clothes and accessories.) Invariably, shopping for Baby becomes a combination of wants and needs. The trick is balancing those without breaking the bank.

There are so many stores hawking crazy-cute baby stuff that an entire book could be dedicated to the best places to shop. But for the sake of space and your bank account I've listed only a smattering of favorites, from cheap and practical to fantastically frivolous. Before you browse, you might want to check out the tips in Chapter 14.

One-Stop Baby Gear Shops

You can buy online from all of the following sources, but you should also be able to find retail locations for most of them near you. For a list of what I consider nursery must-haves, turn to page 192.

Amazon.com
www.amazon.com

This online jungle of retail opportunity gives you reason to spend hours debating over something as simple as a diaper bag—last time I checked they were one shy of 1,000 offerings. Its link to BabiesRUs.com means you can also comparison-shop for strollers, car seats, furniture, clothing, toys, books, and other industry standards. You won't find the cheapest prices here, but you will discover valuable customer reviews on practically every product they sell, deep discounts on classic bedtime books and CDs, free shipping opportunities, and easy online baby-shower registry.

Babies R Us
www.babiesrus.com

Bounce over to this national chain for virtually everything your new child could possibly need. Diapers, diaper pails, swings, clothing, shoes, an astounding assortment of toys—they've got it all. A mommy friend even mentioned she found organic baby food at a fraction of the regular price. Their in-store sales are usually steals. Another bonus: They have an online baby registry.

Bliss Living
www.blissliving.com

This site has all kinds of great unique stuff, from celebrity-preferred diaper bags to custom mommy and daddy jewelry. Especially cool is the array of distinctive hanging letters for spelling your baby's name on the nursery wall.

Burlington Coat Factory
www.burlingtoncoatfactory.com

This discount store's Baby Depot is a good source for inexpensive baby clothing and nursery furniture. During a recent peek at their online shop most changing tables were less than $100. They also had zip-up footie PJs, which were essentially all my kid wore for the first year of her life. One Coat Factory fan from the menagerie pointed out that they don't seem to have the backorder problems that plague many furniture suppliers.

CraigsList
www.craigslist.com

Convenience and great prices are the number-one reasons mommies buy and sell on this community-centric site. Virtually everything you can think of is available here—clothing, cribs, exersaucers, rockers, strollers, you name it—provided you're willing to pick your purchase up from the seller. Busy mommies sometimes sell all their outgrown gear as a bulk purchase, so you may be able to pick up almost everything you need from one source.

Ebay.com

Great deals can be found on eBay, but shipping charges can turn a bargain into a financial burden, and if you don't like your purchase you have no choice but to lump it.

Giggle
www.egiggle.com

Uptown and upscale, this boutique chain and website hand-selects the coolest and highest quality stuff for the baby's bed, bath, body, nursery, and more. Far more expensive than the budget benchmark of Target, but not entirely unapproachable, it's a good happy medium with plenty of stuff in all price ranges—including good "green" products—which is why I registered here (and at Target and Babies R Us) for my shower.

Target
www.target.com

A godsend for the expecting mommy, this cheap national chain has it all—gear, clothing, furniture, and toys. You'll find more furnishings online than you will in a retail outlet, but buyer beware: the chest of drawers I bought online arrived damaged twice and required lots of assembly. (They did give me a substantial discount to deal with it myself and 19 months later it's still going strong, so in the end it was worth it.) Still, if you don't want to spend wads of dough, some inexpensive stuff may be just the ticket. Stop in a nearby store and do a drive-by for all the basics, including onesies, nail clippers, monitors, bathtubs, and more. You can also craft a baby registry on their website.

Online Discounts
You can save tons of money on little- and big-ticket baby items by comparison shopping online. I saved $75 on our car seat alone— and got it from a reputable online dealer. It may take a little research to find the best deals, but if you're counting your coins and can wait for products to be shipped to you, it's definitely time well spent.

Baby Clothing

Also see the stores listed in "One-Stop Baby Gear Shops" starting on page 189.

Also see the stores listed in "One-Stop Baby Gear Shops" starting on page 189.

Baby Gap

www.babygap.com

A fine source for fashioning your favorite new member of the family, this subset of the national clothing chain focuses on classics for the mini him and her. Prices aren't as painless as Old Navy or Target, but the garb tends to be well made and sales items can be great values.

Gymboree

www.gymboree.com

Comparable to the Gap but a little more youthful in style and patterns, this one-stop-fashion shop regularly has a vast selection and fantastic in-store sales. A particularly observant member of the Mommy Menagerie noted that these clothes tend to be very durable.

Janie and Jack

www.janieandjack.com

Yes, it's expensive, but if you're up for splurging on Baby's first wardrobe and prefer classic and preppy styles, this upscale sister to Gymboree (see above) is a good place to do it. But fair warning: some of the stuff is so cute (and regularly on sale) you might be inclined to buy beyond your needs or knowledge. Case in point: Before my daughter was born I bought a 0-3 month halter top and a sweet 12-month white knit sweater. But it turned out I was far too afraid of sunburn to let her hang in a spaghetti-strap cami no matter how cute it was, and by the time the sweater fit her frame, it didn't fit her personality.

Lucky Me

www.luckyme.com

One piece of their handmade knitwear can cost about as much as a night's stay in a fine hotel, but if you have a rich aunt who wants to bless your baby with a special garment or blanket, one of the classic beauties sold through this site will definitely fit the bill. Be warned: Prices are listed in the British pound, which means you'll need to find an online money converter to know the price in U.S. dollars.

The Retro Baby

www.theretrobaby.com

The too-cool-for-school baby will want to shop here for fun onesies and T-shirts with silly slogans like "My mom is the bomb" and "My dad is rad."

Erika's Top 10 Must-Haves

Let's be honest: We don't need half of the stuff we buy to care for a new baby. But if time was money yesterday, today convenience is cash. The items that top my must-have list may not be obvious necessities, but they made life easier and more comfortable, and every mom could use a little of that.

1. Bassinette
Keeping Viva shacked up in an elevated basket next to me stopped me from having to get out of bed to make sure she was still alive, grab her to nurse, or worry that I'd roll over onto her while sleeping.

2. Boppy pillow
If you think pregnancy is bad on your back, wait until you're leaning forward with tensed shoulders and engorged breasts. The boppy elevates the baby so you two can meet in the middle.

3. Bottle warmer
Nothing can warm cold milk or formula fast enough when your kid is crying with hunger. But bottle warmers are as good as it gets. (Use glass bottles or containers.)

4. Bouncy seat
This seat may have seriously been the key to my sanity during the first few months.

5. Breast pump
This wasn't merely handy because I had occasional all-day business meetings, it also gave Colie an opportunity to feed—and be closer to—the baby. Save cash by buying it online.

6. Flannel baby blankets
Viva demanded to sleep swaddled for the first six months of her life. These blankets were the only ones that were sturdy enough to keep her snuggled.

7. Glider
I couldn't fathom spending a big chunk of change on furniture I would normally never buy in a million years, but our glider has been a special seat since the first days of nursing to tonight's bedtime books.

8. Infant car seat and stroller system
I started with a convertible-style car seat. I pulled my sleeping newborn out of her seat to grocery shop exactly one time before replacing it with the snap-and-go type of stroller system.

9. Swing
When Viva's interest in the bouncy seat waned, the swing became the naptime savior.

10. Zip-up PJs
What I wanted was comfy clothing that required as little baby wrangling as possible. Once Viva was out of the newborn stage, Carter's one-piece fleece footie pajamas were the best—and available for under $10 at Costco.

Sckoon
www.sckoon.com

If you're all about organics you can pass the environmentally minded torch to your tot with the adorable 100% organic cotton outfits sold here. You shouldn't be too surprised by the prices. As usual with most organic things these days, you have to pay to play.

Tutti Bella
www.tuttibella.com

If you have the funds and the gumption to dress your little dame or dude in the trendiest, most fabulous clothes, go directly to this website. The European and American fashions found here are fierce and sophisticated, just like their price tags. You'll also find "it" diaper bags, glamorous baby blankets, and bedding. The fact that they offer a three-level Frequent Buyer Program should give you an idea of just how addictive shopping for Baby can be.

Baby Furnishings
Also see stores listed in "One-Stop Baby Gear Shops."

Baby Geared
www.babygeared.com

Modernist mommies with megabucks should point their mice to this chic shop selling the hippest baby furniture around. As for the rest of us, at least we can dream. Check out the awe-inspiring highchairs and corresponding prices, both of which might make your jaw drop. You'll find sensational-looking sleep sacks here, too—at twice the price of regular fleece or cotton varieties.

Modern Seed
www.modernseed.com

For the chic furniture-fanatic mommy-to-be, this site is more of a tease than a big hunk of chocolate cake—especially considering the grown-up prices for the likes of Eames storage units and Stokke cribs. At least they have a gift registry; if there's something you just have to have, perhaps your pals can ante up for the best group gift ever.

Pottery Barn Kids
www.potterybarnkids.com

Quintessentially adorable interiors don't come cheaply at this offshoot of the ubiquitous home store chain, but if you simply must have your child's name spelled out in block letters on the nursery wall, are looking for fabulous traditional furnishings, or need a fuzzy pink or blue bassinet bedding set you'll find it—and a lot more—here. And yes, they have a registry, so ideally someone else can pick up the tab for the perfect changing table.

My birthing plan was pretty simple. I intended to try getting through the whole shebang without medication, but was very open to changing my mind at any given time. I was anti-episiotomy (an incision of the perineum to widen the baby's escape route), pro-husband in the room, and not sure how I would feel about my mother's greatly desired presence. I told mom up front that she was welcome to hang at the hospital but might or might not witness the birth. Colie and I agreed that he would cut the umbilical cord and made a list of people to call after the baby was born, and that was pretty much that.

As short as it was, my plan didn't go as expected. I went into labor four days past my due date at around 3:30 in the afternoon. It didn't start with a feeling, but with "bloody show"— ruddy-brown underwear evidence that the mucus plug was unplugging. I gave the hospital and my husband a heads-up and spent the next five hours lounging on the couch, eating soup, watching TV, and charting the contraction times and durations with Colie, who left work the second he heard the news.

When the contractions were seven minutes apart and about fifty seconds in duration they were still no more bothersome than an everyday menstrual cramp. Still, we set off for the hospital on their recommendation because we lived an hour away and I was GBS positive (a carrier of the Group B strep virus, which is common), which meant the hospital wanted to introduce antibiotics to ensure I couldn't pass the bacteria to the baby.

I waddled into admitting at around 9:30pm. They examined me, learned that my water still hadn't broken, saw that I was only two centimeters dilated, and sent me home, recommending I return when my contractions had been one minute long and three minutes apart for at least one hour.

Rather than drive all the way home, we went to my mother's place 10 minutes away. I had long wanted Colie to watch the movie "The Sure Thing," so I popped it in the DVD player and figured I'd pass the time with a lighthearted comedy. But within 20 minutes the contractions were no laughing matter, although to say it was uncomfortable would be a joke. At first, labor was a crazy, jump-out-of-my-skin kind of pain—especially because I had yet to learn that the best way to beat contractions was to join them. Lacking the comforts of home probably made matters worse. I anxiously counted down the moments until I could return to the hospital and fled for the car a good 10 minutes before I'd reached the nurse's one-hour goal. When I returned to the hospital just before midnight, I learned that my dilation hadn't progressed. But the pain definitely had. As each wave crashed upon me I doubled over, unable to speak or move. During the three minutes between each one, I was either trying to describe a contraction (which was and still is impossible), dry heaving (very normal), or waddling to the check-in area's bathroom with Colie's help. A bowel movement during one of those trips had me slouched over on the toilet, humiliated, and whining to my calm and supportive husband, who had never before witnessed me make a donation to the porcelain foundation, "All modesty is lost now." Ironically, both of us remember that moment with deep fondness. It took being a toilet invalid to remind me that revealing our true, unedited, and most vulnerable selves really is the thing that bonds two people together.

Two hours later my stubborn cervix was still ironclad. I was less sturdy. I had

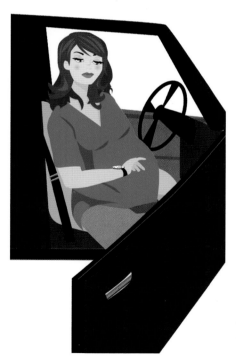

two choices: To go wait it out on mom's uncomfortable couch or to check in and allow the hospital to expedite my labor. At that moment comfort trumped everything, so I took my first step in abandoning my birthing plan. At about 1am, I agreed to be induced through a drug called oxytocin (aka Pitocin). By 3:30am, I was welcoming the numbing affects of the epidural, which left me about as mobile as a Sunday night rump roast. The rest was a snowball of medications and procedures. The staff broke my water, I was wired up to a fetal monitor and a bunch of bags with drips, and I faded in and out of consciousness— pain-free and brain-free.

Early the next afternoon when my cervix was still at a snug four centimeters and my daughter's heart rate was periodically dropping, I was informed that the next step was a C-section. Since my doctor was on vacation I had to wait several hours before a doctor I'd never met, who turned out to be perfectly lovely, was available to perform my operation.

By 3:30pm I was in surgery, accompanied by my husband and mom draped in blue scrubs. A low curtain blocked my view of the surgeons cutting a small incision at my bikini line and pulling out and setting aside a few organs to get at my girl. But it did not shield me from joining them in a casual mid-surgery discussion of good ways to cook fish. (Yes, really.) Viva was born at 3:59pm, about 24 hours after our adventure began. Her umbilical cord was wrapped around her neck, which is apparently more common and less threatening than you might think. She weighed 7 pounds, 3.5 ounces, and was a strapping 20 inches in length.

Colie cut the cord and they put my daughter up to my face so that I could meet her. I had to concentrate to stop my eyes from crossing due to the drugs, but I remember that moment with great clarity. It was one of the most powerful, deeply emotional events of my life.

After a quick patch-up job on my incision, we were all in the recovery room and then in a hospital room where our new threesome shacked up for four days.

No, my birthing plan did not go as expected. But it did have some perks: We loved staying in the hospital for the first days. It was like being at a hotel with round-the-clock baby training and services. By the time we left, my milk had come in so I didn't have to anxiously wait without professional support and reassurance. And we had enough schooling to feel confident in our parenting abilities.

I never paid enough attention to the details of cesarean sections to know they are major surgeries that include long and painful recoveries, so the next several weeks had some unexpected challenges. But you know what? None of it mattered. Not the pain of labor, nor the disappointment of not having a baby the way we'd planned, or even the excruciating pain in my gut that occurred for several weeks afterward whenever I sneezed, laughed, or tried to get out of bed. At the time it was powerful, overwhelming, emotional, and yes, painful. But even at my darkest moments it was also a glorious day that produced a bonding moment in the bathroom, tales to tell, and the greatest joy of my life.

THE READY OR NOT: PREPARING FOR THE BIG DAY AND BEYOND

Frankly, I don't think it's possible to be truly ready for the next phase, unless you are already a mommy and know the drill. However you slice it, the transition is that dramatic. But you can make the change easier by planning ahead and stocking up on essentials. Take a peek here for fast information on how to prepare for the delivery-room dash, the gear you'll need for your newborn, and must-have new mommy equipment.

Pre-Baby Prep

Some preparatory actions are more important than others. The baby's room is a good example. While you may want the nursery painted a pretty color, decorated with adorable baby artwork, and dangling with fun mobiles, the only things your little one will see when it's born are items within six inches of his eyes—and I'll bet his preference would be a nice big boob and his parents' smiling faces. While I wholeheartedly encourage you to have your whimsical way with the baby room, there are more important preparations at hand. Read on for tips, must-dos, and must-buys; consider yourself prepared, and look at the rest as icing on your newborn's birthday cake.

Take birthing and newborn classes.

These brief courses tend to be held by hospitals, independent education companies, and experts-for-hire and are generally advised for expecting parents that are headed into the homestretch (think seven to nine months along). Usually held over a weekend or several evenings, they offer extensive and extremely helpful details and tips on birthing choices, how to prepare for labor and delivery, possible birthing scenarios, newborn care, nursing, CPR, and even things as basic as how to bathe a new baby. They are also good places to network with other expecting parents and learn about local resources for pediatricians, baby stores, childcare, and anything else you might want to know.

Even if you know the drill, attending a class can be very helpful, especially if you want to get your partner more involved, educated, and prepared to help you deal with labor. Classes usually follow one school of birthing thought (think Lamaze, Bradley, or hypnobirthing) or a combination of methods. If you don't know which type suits you, visit page 240 for online resources describing each style.

To find good classes in your area, ask your mommy friends or practitioner. Also, if you want a less-biased view on current medical practices, trends, and your birthing options, take a class from an independent instructor rather than at a hospital.

Create a birthing plan.

A birthing plan is just that—a plan. Like a vacation itinerary, it should list the details and order in which you want things to happen, from the minute you feel that first contraction until that wrinkly little ball of joy is safely shoved into your arms. I'm not talking the amount of times you expect to scream at your husband, "Don't touch me!" or "Shut up!" during labor. There are more

> ### False Starts
> Women who arrive at hospitals thinking they are ready to deliver are regularly told to go home and wait until they're further dilated.

important considerations to take into account, including whether you're down with drugs, who you want in the room with you, your position on episiotomies, who cuts the umbilical cord, what you want to happen immediately after your infant is born, and who will water the plants or feed and walk the dog if you end up staying away from home longer than expected.

A birthing class and your practitioner can clue you in to a lot of these choices, but you can also read up on them. (See page 238 for information on worthy books and websites.) Review your decisions with your practitioner and partner, but also write them on paper, bring copies to your birthing destination, and give one to the staff when you check in.

Regardless of whether your plan is a sentence or a 10-page script, a birthing plan is still nothing more than an outline of how you'd like things to go down. Just like vacation itineraries, they are subject to change at any given moment due to acts of God, your own whims, or unforeseen dilemmas. For that reason your plan should include a "Go with the Flow" clause, which essentially means that if your birth takes an unexpected and necessary turn, you will relax and remember that the ultimate goal of all birth plans is a healthy baby and healthy mom. How you get there isn't nearly as important.

Read up on and practice labor-coping strategies.

Even if you plan on getting doped up the second you waddle into the hospital, you would be wise to brush up on the art of managing labor pain. Good breathing exercises did me a world of good when I finally gave in to the notion of numbness and then had to wait for more than an hour for the overbooked anesthesiologist. Relaxation techniques would have been just as handy had we stumbled upon a rogue traffic jam en route to our birthing destination. There are numerous methods for natural pain management, most of which can be explored online or through books. For more details, see page 238.

The Mommy Menagerie On
...Did your water break on its own?

Just how likely is it that you'll experience a surprise flash flood before labor begins? If you look at the percentages of 98 menagerie pregnancies, it's anybody's guess.

53% of pregnancies kicked off their finale with an unsolicited water break.

47% of mommies-to-be had a professional break their bag for them.

If you're planning to breastfeed, do some research.

I'll bet you're wondering, "Why research nursing? Isn't it as easy as sticking a nipple in a baby's mouth?" The answer is yes and no. For many mommies, including me, nursing was the most stressful part of new motherhood. It wasn't the traumatizing rite of passage of waiting a few days for my milk to come in while I imagined that my child was wailing with hunger that really sucked (pardon the pun); it wasn't the painful transition into a breastfeeding routine, which included cracked and bleeding nipples that caused me grief; my problem was that after a few months of smooth sailing, I was not producing enough milk to keep my kid sated.

One thing I can tell you is that you do not want to begin researching troubleshooting tactics when you really need them. I can honestly say I've never felt more desperate. For books and websites dedicated to the subject, see page 244.

Start shopping.

There are a gazillion things that books, websites, and mommies recommend you buy for the baby or yourself that you actually don't need for the first several weeks, if at all. But there are just as many modern must-haves that you'll probably want to stock up on before you go into labor. For a complete list of essentials, see "The New Baby Starter Kit" on page 209, make your shopping list, beg for and borrow everything you can, and get ready to give your credit card a good workout. But consider the following shopping tips before you get going.

Welcome hand-me-downs. Most moms want to put their brand new baby into a smart new outfit. But shortly afterward, many of them—myself included—are perfectly happy slipping their kids into pre-worn stuff— especially in the beginning when outfits are obsolete after one or two appearances. This goes for gear, toys, and everything else, too.

Shop sparingly for clothing. Don't buy larger sizes too far in advance. Just because you find a fabulous swimsuit in size 12 to 18 months doesn't mean your baby will fit into it in time for your summer vacation. My tall and lean little one was wearing three to six month-size tops when she was a year old, and two of my all-time favorite splurge outfits that I bought a year in advance were worn exactly once before they were outgrown.

Size isn't the only variable. Personalities play a part, too. Before Viva was born, I dreamed of dressing her in chic outfits. But I quickly found I was too cheap to pay full price, too lazy to scout sales, and too practical to bother with little buttons when there is a whole world of one-zipper jimmies and simple-snap rompers. Simultaneously, Viva showed she wasn't the frilly dress type when she started walking at 10 months, digging in the dirt, eating sand, and bathing herself (and any clothes she's wearing) whenever any water was in reach. Alas, all of the fabulous clothing I bought for her in advance essentially became closet art.

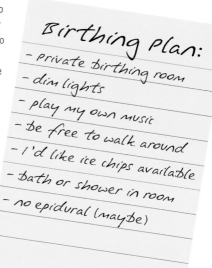

Birthing Plan:
- private birthing room
- dim lights
- play my own music
- be free to walk around
- I'd like ice chips available
- bath or shower in room
- no epidural (maybe)

Get your car seat and have it installed.

Babies don't pop out on cue like showgirls in giant birthday cakes. However, they can be an equally startling—and scantily clad—surprise to the recipient. At least three menagerie members received knocks at their uterine doors a solid six weeks before their permanent houseguest was expected. For this reason it's important to get your driving ducks in a row, especially because, although you can get by for your first days without most of the baby baubles, you cannot legally drive your darling home from her birthplace until she is safely strapped into a rear-facing car seat.

Once you've purchased a seat, call your local police department to get it installed; they are likely to have a program that allows you to bring your seat in for free installation or that sends a trained officer to your house to help you hook it up. At a minimum they will direct you to a center that will ensure your seat is properly installed. For seat-selection tips, check out the shopping list on page 222.

> **Fill Your Gas Tank**
>
> If you will use your car to get to the place you intend to give birth, keep it filled with gas as your due date nears. You definitely don't want to have to wait at the pump when you're about to pop.

Get a pediatrician.

If you give birth in a hospital, you will be required to provide the staff with the contact information of your child's pediatrician before you leave, which essentially means you'd better find one now. If you're not sure how to go about it, ask your practitioner or mommy friends for recommendations and interview your options.

Keep in mind that there is more to a good doctor than competence, a license, and a friendly bedside manner. Their after-hours program, for one. I didn't inquire in advance about my pediatrician's late-night logistics and was referred to a basic hotline and charged $10 per call the first time I called (and called and called). Trust me: This is not something you want to find out during your first string of panicked midnight calls.

> **Call Your Practitioner**
>
> When you go into labor or your water breaks, contact your provider and review the next steps.

Make a list of emergency numbers.

If you take a birthing class you may receive a sheet of local resources, but regardless, you should draft and post in your home a list of critical phone numbers. Include poison control (which I just called last week when Viva snuck a fresh snack from the cat box), your pediatrician, pediatric after-hours number, helpful family members, and anyone else you, your partner, or any childcare provider might need to contact in case of emergency. If you're nursing, add contacts for local breastfeeding support groups and lactation consultants. While you're at it, you might as well post a sheet with infant CPR instructions and diagrams, too.

Research all of your home-delivery options.

Soon the days of dashing out to run an errand, grab dinner or a video, or buy diapers will be about as leisurely as climbing Mount Everest. Luckily, more and more companies offer home delivery. When I was holed up with a newborn, I relied on my local grocer (which I learned delivered for a small fee), counted on netflix.com for a continual stream of DVDs, called on a barrage of restaurants that delivered, and fell in love with 1800diapers.com, which offers cheap prices on disposable diapers and fast, free door-to-door service. Think of the things that you'd like brought to you and research delivery options.

Secure helping hands if you can.

The first weeks of parenthood are surprising, exhausting, and transitional to say the least. The last thing you need is to worry about doing laundry or getting dinner on the table. If you have family or friends that are willing to help you with housework, rock the baby while you snag a shower or run errands, enlist them beforehand. But also give yourself an out just in case you're in no mood for visitors. Equally important is to politely decline offers from anyone who has a history of driving you crazy.

One member of the menagerie recommends lining up a post-partum doula. She explained, "I spent so much time preparing for the delivery that I didn't even consider how overwhelmed we'd be when we brought the little one home. I got help within the week and that saved my sanity. She did anything I wanted and I could ask her to do things that you might not want to ask your mom or mother-in-law."

Start thinking about childcare, if you will need it.

If you're going to stay home and care for your tot, more power to ya. But if you've got to or want to return to work, you need to come up with a solid childcare plan. In fact, as pathetic as it sounds, depending on where you live, you may need to think about childcare even if you intend to wait two or three years—that's how competitive and waitlisted some of today's top pre-preschools and preschools are.

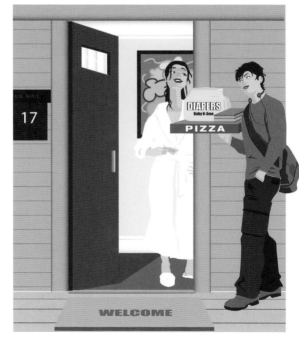

The concept of entrusting my child to a stranger scared the hell out of me, but I found that the sooner I jumped into the process of finding good childcare, the sooner I overcame my deep anxiety about it. In fact, I was completely at ease within five minutes of meeting the woman who I ultimately hired to care for my daughter—and a friend of a friend of a friend discovered her on craigslist.com. It was my first real experience with mother's intuition (and reference checks).

A qualified and loving nanny or daycare center can come from any number of resources. Good starting points include friends, family, local parenting networks, preschools, and agencies (which, alas, charge a premium). When you start interviewing, it is important to ask for references, learn if the person can legally drive and is trained in first aid, and discover her ideas about discipline, to name a few.

Pack a bag.

Because I'm a type-A personality, I had the bag I intended to bring to the hospital packed and in the car weeks before my due date. But even if you're more of a type-ZZZZZ person, it's not a bad idea to load up the luggage with special items you know you are going to want with you while pushing out a baby. (Yes, a hospital or birthing center will provide essentially everything you need, including gowns, panties, and maxi-pads for you and newborn T-shirts, diapers, and caps for your baby. But you may want to bring your own.) Additionally, it's a good idea to pack as little as possible, since you'll have less to keep track of and you may have your hands full toting home a tot and flowers and teddy bears from well-wishers. But if listening to your Yanni CD is an essential part of your birthing plan, the last thing you want to do is chance forgetting it during a mid-labor packing scramble. For a list of what to bring and leave behind, see the "What to Pack Cheat Sheet" on page 206.

Wetting the Bed

When one of my girlfriends told me she ruined her new mattress when her water broke in bed, I instantly dashed to Target and bought a waterproof pad to put under my sheets. I also carried a towel in the car in case of a front-seat flood. My water never broke on its own, but those precautions stopped me from obsessing over the possibility—and thus made them worth the effort. Now we break out the pad when we want to picnic on damp grass.

Pre-register with the hospital.

If you are giving birth in a hospital, you will probably be asked by your physician to pre-register sometime between the end of your seventh and the beginning of your ninth month of pregnancy. If you are not invited, definitely inquire. Trust me: You do not want to hassle with mounds of paperwork between contractions.

Cook and freeze yummy food.

If your friends and family are gracious and knowledgeable, they will shower you with wonderful home-cooked meals the minute you bring your baby home. But don't count on it. Make and freeze readymade meals. Lasagna, enchiladas, and pasta sauce were popular at my house.

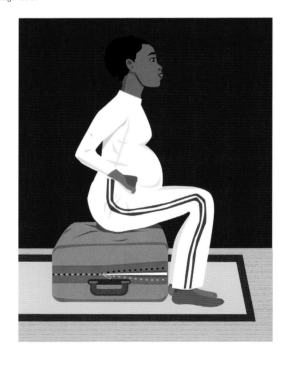

The Mommy Menagerie On ...Did you get an epidural?

To medicate or not to medicate. That was the question. 98 mommies answered.

81% of laboring ladies opted to ease their pain.

19% grinned and bore it.

Get a pedicure.

While it's not required that you have perfectly painted toes when you push out a tot, it is a lot easier to pamper yourself before the big day. Besides, it might be months before you get to a nail salon again.

Clear your calendar.

One surefire way for a new mom to go manic is to over-commit while learning to navigate new motherhood. You may think you'll be up for visits from all of your friends the minute you welcome your child into the world, but better to give yourself the opportunity to decide that once you get there and see what your new world is really like. Warn family and pals that you'll get in touch when you're ready to talk and keep your schedule loose.

Hospital Visits

If you welcome friends and family to visit you in the hospital, tell them to call first. I had a surprise visit from two friends 18 hours after I went into labor, a good six hours before I had my baby. I was drugged out of my mind and bawling because I'd just been informed of my impending c-section. It was not the ideal time to play hostess.

Agree on how to deal with visitors.

I was quite happy to show off my new baby to friends. But I was not so keen on the surprising amount of people who overstayed their welcome. Learn from my mistakes: If you're not blunt enough to wave off loiterers in your living room with a quick, "Thanks for coming, now beat it," come up with an evacuation plan. Blaming Baby is always good. ("Excuse me, I've got to feed the baby and it usually takes two hours.") Or get your partner to do the dirty work. Also, hint hard that preferred guests arrive with a fully prepared meal for hungry parents.

The Mommy Menagerie On ...What did you bring to the hospital or wish you had brought?

Most everyone chimed in on the contents of their birthing bags. Here are some highlights:

"What DIDN'T I pack? We were doing hypno-birth-ing (no meds, using intensive relaxation techniques to cope) so I brought: flameless candles; an electric heat-ing pad; a CD Player with new age CDs (e.g. Enya, Stephen Halpern); a sound machine (e.g. waterfall, ocean, white noise) (USED THIS); an aromatherapy kit; extra pillows (USED THESE); food (I wasn't going to go without!); a nightgown/clothes for after. I don't think I missed anything. The caveat to this is that I labored at home for 22 hours and I used a lot of the things there. But once I got to the hospital, things just got way too intense for me to care about smelling jasmine or being bathed in flickering candlelight."

"Packed the whole car—yoga ball, boom box, CDs, bathing suits (for me and my husband), clothes, toiletries, makeup. Only used toiletries. Had an emergency C-section and all the 'birthing' items never made it out of the car."

"Lip stuff and a headband were great to have. I was happy I had toiletries and lipstick for going home."

"We should have brought a sleeping bag and pad for my husband."

"I probably packed too much, but I did use it all. For me: underwear, nursing bra, nursing pads, Kotex, pajamas and clothes to wear home, hair dryer, curling iron, make-up, toiletries (yes, I did shower, wash, dry, curl my hair, and put on make-up the morning after I had all my kids—even the twins who were a C-section). I also packed magazines, snacks, and my cell phone and camera. For the babies I packed a take-home outfit, blanket, binky, and diaper bag packed with diapers, wipes, burp rags, etc. I can't think of anything I didn't bring that I wish I had since I pretty much packed the whole house."

"Portable CD player with CDs (helpful), a variety of snacks for me and my husband (VERY helpful, especially since the dietary staff was on strike that week), my own pillows from home (very helpful), toiletries (very helpful), thick socks (very helpful), nursing pajamas (did not use), birthing ball (did not use), tennis balls in a sock (did not use). I wish we had brought extra cash hidden in my bag because my husband's wallet was stolen from our room."

"With my second child, I brought a photograph of my first child and displayed it next to my bed. It was great because the nurses didn't treat me like an idiot and my daughter felt special every time she came in to visit me."

"My favorite thing to bring was a new going-home skirt. I knew that I would feel badly wearing a baggy maternity shirt and stretch pants, but I had no idea what shape my body would be in. So, with each of my hospital visits, I bought a new, cute, elastic waistband skirt."

"I wish I had brought my body pillow."

What to Pack Cheat Sheet

Some pregnancy books recommend you lug so many things into the labor and delivery room with you that I packed as though I were heading off for a weeklong vacation. Ironically, the hospital supplied me with all the necessities, so almost everything I brought just became a burden that I had to keep track of. Below are what I consider the real essentials—as well as some items I recommend you skip. Check them out and embellish based on your needs and desires.

 Amusements.
If you're in and out of the hospital you may need nothing, but if you shack up like we did, you'll be happy with an arsenal of distractions, from magazines to a DVD player to a laptop (provided the hospital has internet access).

 Baby blanket.
BYO or depart with at least one from the hospital. I used a rolled-up hospital blanket as a car-seat bumper for baby's bobbling head and draped another blanket over her tiny legs and feet for the ride home.

 Baby outfit.
Bring one for the ride home. Make sure it's warm and cozy and has legs so that you can use the car seat harness properly.

 Birthing plan.
If you've got it, check-in is the time to flaunt it. Give an extra to your partner or coach for instant reference.

 Breast pads.
Buy and bring disposables to see if you need to use them before investing in washable cotton versions. Mine are still in the box.

 Boppy or other nursing pillow.
I wish I had this menagerie member recommendation when I went to the hospital. Nursing a newborn on pillows is a precarious proposition.

 Camera, camcorder, or both.
During this adventure a picture really is worth a million words.

 Camera or camcorder charger or both.
You will kick yourself forever if your batteries die and cannot be revived.

 Cell phone.
A must have for obvious reasons (although some hospitals may prohibit their use).

 Cell phone charger.
This is one time you really don't want your batteries to die.

 Changes of clothes for partner or coach.
Pack extra. Colie and I planned to pop in and out of the hospital. He was there for five days with only one change of clothes.

Cosmetics.
Depends on whether you have guests, which you may not know until you find out how long you will have to stay. Pack only what you would absolutely want if you were receiving visitors.

 Glasses, contact lenses and supplies, or both.
If you need them, definitely bring them.

 Hard candies.
I didn't use them to keep my laboring mouth moist, but many menagerie members did. Some labor and delivery units won't allow them, so check with your practitioner.

 Headband or ponytail holders.
Anything to make hair mainte-nance easier is a plus in my book.

 Health insurance card.
You will need this. Have it handy.

 Lip balm.
Yes, yes, and yes. Pack three and put them where you know you can find them.

 List of names and phone numbers of people to call.
You'll definitely want this.

 A loose-fitting outfit for the ride home.
Don't go dreaming that you'll push that baby out and pop back into your pre-pregnancy slacks. You will still be huge, so pack like it.

 Music.
I didn't use or wish I had a boom box and I was in the hospital for five days.

 Nightgowns.
Skip 'em. Hospital gowns are free, provide easy access for bathroom breaks, and won't stress you out when you stain them with inevitable yoohoo leakage.

 Nursing bra.
Bring one unless you want to hang loose for visiting friends and family.

 Oil for massage.
I don't know anyone who brought this and used this, although I'm sure there are some advocates out there.

 Pencil or pen and pad.
Brilliant idea. You will use it to remind yourself of a gazillion things after the baby is born, from phone calls you need to return to a list of people to thank for sending flowers to your room.

What to Pack continued

 Pillows with brightly colored pillowcases.
It is nice to have your favorite pillows from home, and your partner may enjoy using them too. Colorful covers stop the hospital from mistakenly claiming them.

 Rear-facing car seat.
You can't leave the hospital without this.

 Robe.
Go for it if you wish. It's nice to stroll in something snuggly. I didn't bring one and didn't much miss it, but then again I'm the type who doesn't flinch at wandering the hospital halls with my hiney peeking out.

 Sanitary napkins.
Forget 'em. They will be provided for you.

 Slippers with non-slip soles.
Bring 'em. The hospital will give you socks for strolling, but they're hardly plush.

 Snacks.
My birthing location had all the snacks I needed, but I wasn't allowed to eat until I detoxed. Find out your situation and pack accordingly.

 Snacks and beverages for partner.
It's important that your partner stay energized during your labor without having to dash down the road for some fast-food. Handy snacks and hydrating beverages will help.

 Socks.
I loved wearing my own thick fluffy pairs, especially when my body was cold while I was coming off of the drugs.

 Toiletries.
Go light. All you really need is a toothbrush, toothpaste, deodorant, your favorite soap, shampoo, conditioner, lotion, and a comb or brush.

 Toiletries for partner.
Definitely have him lug his necessary gear.

 Underwear.
Leave your lovelies at home and stick with the provided disposable mesh stuff. Ask the staff for some for the road, too. Recovery is messy business.

 A watch with second hand to time contractions.
Skip it. Hospital rooms have huge clocks with second hands.

The New Baby Starter Kit

Menagerie member Brigette Miller is the kind of mommy every pregnant woman should have in her back pocket. A friend of a friend of a friend and a mother of two, she not only diligently filled out my laborious pregnancy questionnaire, but also forwarded an absolutely brilliant manifesto of what you should buy and what you should skip when preparing for motherhood. It was so concise, complete, and right-on that when I sat down to write this section I e-mailed Brigette and asked if she minded if I combined her comments with mine and included them in this book. She generously agreed. It's worth noting that if you can't or don't want to buy everything on this list, you will still easily be able to raise a happy, healthy child. A lot of this stuff is convenience for parents, but not absolutely critical for Baby. Without further ado here it is: The straight scoop on what you may or may not need or want.

Private Room Rates

If you want a private post-partum room, request it at the time of admission. But know that you might have to pay extra for it.

Diapering

Contrary to many parents, I enjoy changing diapers. It's the one activity where I have my squirmy girl's full attention, can kiss her feet, blow on her belly, sing songs, and care for her in a way that she will soon never need again. She's at an age now where protest is part of the routine, but it's still a sweet exchange—especially when I have all of the essentials organized and well stocked. Whether you revel in the ritual or not, you definitely need the following items.

Diapers. I'm not going to tell you which type of diaper to use—with a little research you can decide whether cloth or disposable is ideal for you. What I will say, however, is that you'll need at least 200 on hand, because the only things that will be more intimate than you with your newborn's digestive downloads are the 100 or so diapers you'll go through in the first week alone. If, by some chance, you don't use them, you can return them for the next size up. You might also want to stock up on two different sizes—newborn and size 1— because a large baby will quickly transition from the starter size, if not go directly to them. Even if that's not the case, you're ahead of the game when you need to trade up. Equally important if you're doing disposables is not to buy too many; some diapers will fit your baby better than others, and you are likely to become loyal to the brand that doesn't force you to regularly change pee-dampened pants. Once you commit, check 1800diapers.com for great prices and free delivery. For starters, try Brigette's and my favorite: Pampers Swaddlers. They are very luxurious and plush.

"If you can't buy every-thing, you will still raise a happy, healthy child."

Wipes. There's no way around using tons of these handy booty buffers. But not all of them are created equal. For Baby's first months when skin is ultrasensitive, skip wet wipes altogether and use soft, dry cotton wetted with water. I loved the velvety four-inch cotton gauze squares sold at San Francisco's Day One baby center. They source them from a medical-supply company and sell a pack of 200 for $6.95—and they will ship them to you if you don't live nearby. If you're interested, call 415-440-3291 and buy at least six packs; stuck in your diaper bag, they'll also be useful for swabbing spit-up and other rogue liquids. Later-on bets for Baby's sensitive skin are alcohol- and fragrance-free wet wipes, which can be bought in bulk from discount stores or 1800diapers.com. Buy more than you think you'll need; for at least the next two years there will be no such thing as too many wipes.

Diaper bag. Truth is, you can easily get by carrying baby essentials in any big bag. But I found value in purchasing a designated diaper bag for a few reasons. First, because we had a specific bag for baby stuff, we kept all the essentials in it and knew where they were at all times. Second, it was unisex enough that it didn't emasculate my husband when he carried it (although Colie is so nonchalant he wouldn't have cared if it were hot pink faux fur). Third, since it's not one of my coveted purses I don't care when it gets dirty or barfed on. Fourth, it has compartments that are hard for my daughter to infiltrate, which is important when I'm carrying things I don't want her to promptly stick into her mouth. Finally, it was an excuse to buy a new accessory—and what's not to like about that?

Diaper pail. A diaper pail is just a glorified trashcan with a tightly sealing lid. Its one true benefit is that it lessens the odor of used diapers stuck within them. But that luxury will cost you repeatedly since most pails require you to purchase and use pricy refill liners. As a selective cheapskate I loathe buying liners and repeatedly take operational shortcuts with my pail, which results in a detectable diaper odor after all. Now my pail is in the bathroom next to my daughter's room and I transport dirty diapers there several times a day. If you're a spendthrift like me, you can go with a cute garbage can or find a happy medium with a pail called the Diaper Champ, which seals like the fancy pails but uses regular garbage bags.

Diaper-rash ointment. Before Viva was born, I loaded up on organic health-food-store diaper creams, but the second our daughter got her first serious rash they couldn't begin to curb our poor girl's blistering sores. (FYI: At its worst, diaper rash can be quite gory.) I immediately turned to the hard-core, over-the-counter drugstore stuff and found it to be far more effective. My best bet for really tough rashes is as much naked time as possible (for Viva, not me) and Desitin or A&D topped with a hearty sprinkle of everyday cornstarch. (Brigette loves A&D in the pump.)

One tip for the road: If and when your baby has a rash and is a little older, ALWAYS rinse wipes thoroughly in warm water before using them because unrinsed wipes can sting Baby's already suffering skin.

> ## Stocking the Diaper Bag
>
> Stock your diaper bag with absolute essentials: several diapers, a small container of wet wipes, diaper cream, and a changing pad or liner for public changing tables and other surfaces. Also include a complete change of baby clothes—trust me, you WILL need it— a burp cloth, toys, a pacifier if your baby uses one, and a backup bottle of milk or formula, if applicable. Also, always restock the bag the second you get home so that when you are in a harried dash to get out of the house again you don't forget anything.

Disposable changing-table liners. One of my wisest new-mom investments, disposable liners have a soft cotton front and a thin waterproof back. Place them atop your changing pad so when a flash flood hits you won't have to immediately do laundry. Also stick some in your diaper bag for the inevitable day when you have to change your child on the counter of a public restroom or in the backseat of your car. You can find them online or order them from San Francisco's Day One baby center at 415-440-3291.

Clothing & Blankets

You should have a starter wardrobe worked out before you bring Baby home. But you may need less than you think. Read the following tips and shopping list before you buy. Then put the money you save skipping pointless purchases toward a much-deserved postpartum outfit or massage.

Disposable Diaper Deals

I use www.1800diapers.com more than any other site because there is no such thing as enough diapers and baby wipes. I'd rather spend my time doing something other than shopping for them, and all the big brands of disposables—including the most PC brand Seventh Generation—are sold very cheaply and in bulk here, along with bulk boxes of wipes. The clincher, however, is speedy free delivery. Get friends to start buying from the site and you'll score additional discounts, too.

Bibs. No, your new baby isn't going to sit down at the dinner table anytime soon, but for the next several months she is likely to spit up nearly as much liquid as she swallows, drool, and occasionally be a veritable fountain of fun. Breaking out a bib can stop Baby from having to do three or more costume changes in one day. (You, on the other hand, are destined to rock the regurgitated look even if you carry burp cloths, as babies are very good at surprise projectile attacks.) Skip bibs with Velcro. Look for snaps and buy two or three.

Booties or socks. Most mommies I know consider baby socks a pointless expense since they never seem to stay on. But other mommies love them. Those that do, stand by The Gap's bootie socks, which come in six-packs and have little rubber grips on the bottom. Buy one pack and see where you stand.

Gowns. These soft, warm dresses that gather at the bottom are great for bedtime (aka all the time), even for boy babies. Because they're elastic at the bottom, rather than snapped, they make changing a sleepy baby really easy. They are also good for newborns because they are comfy and warm without being too binding. Three should do you.

> "put the money you save skipping purchases toward a postpartum outfit."

The Mommy Menagerie On ...The Top 10 Must-Haves When You Get Home From the Hospital

97 mommies chimed in on the most useful and essential items to have on hand when bringing Baby home. See if you've got their goods on your shopping list.

1. Diapers
Given the amount of these poop-catching pouches you will go through in your child's first days, never mind his or her first two years, it's no surprise that these everyday essentials topped the charts with 36% of the vote.

2. Blankets
Whether they were described as swaddling, receiving, or just big, snuggly blankets, 33% of mommies warmed up to the idea of nice thick wraps for their beloved little burritos.

3. Bassinette, Moses Basket, or Cradle
There's nothing wrong with Baby going direct to a crib, but 20% of mommies considered a more moderate-size training bed a must-have.

4. Prepared Foods
New parents rarely find time to do more than reheat and regroup. For this reason 18% of mommies cooked up the idea of stocking the fridge and cupboards with easy edibles, such as readymade foods, frozen homemade or store-bought meals, and healthy snacks.

5. Breast Pump
16% of mommies migrated toward this manmade milking system for reasons such as jumpstarting the flow, offering up a bottle of fresh stuff to a preemie with baby-latching trouble, and relieving over-engorgement.

6. Wipes
The yin to the diaper's yang, these handy disposable cloths were surely on every mommy's shopping list, but 13% of them made a point of mentioning them.

7. Nursing Pads a.k.a. Breast Pads
Like pasties minus the sequins and adhesive, these padded cotton nipple covers block blouses from lactation leaks and found fans in 12% of the menagerie.

8. Onesies
11% of mommies mentioned these cute little legless unitards that snap in the crotch.

9. Help, Bouncy Seat, and Burp Cloths
Topping the essentials list for 10% of mommies was aid from mom, a friend, nanny, doula or anyone else who can pick up some slack during the first days of parenthood. Tied for ninth place were the lifesaving bouncy seat with vibrate mode and burp cloths, which are ideal for wiping up spit, pee, milk, and all kinds of other fun fluids that are about to come your way.

10. Sleep Sacks
9% of mommies cuddled up to this genius invention, which is essentially a tiny zip-up sleeping bag with holes for your little one's head and arms.

Hats. Your instincts to keep Baby's head covered are right; unless it's really hot outside or inside your house, it's recommended that you keep your newborn's head cozy and warm with a light cap, even indoors. You'll get a freebie from the hospital, so two tête-toppers are enough. Add one brimmed hat for sunny outings with Baby, and if you have a winter baby and live in a cool climate, get a thicker cap, too.

Homecoming outfit. Not knowing how freaked out I would be to dress up my wrinkly, red, and astoundingly floppy newborn, I brought a cute and cuddly homecoming outfit to the hospital—with pantlegs so I could properly strap her into the car seat. Were I to do it over again I'd forget fashion and go with ease of use. Whatever you decide to do, consider getting a "preemie" size outfit, as it's about the only thing that will fit properly. Brigette's son, who was 9 pounds, 8 ounces at birth, wore preemie sizes for the first three weeks. Come to think of it, 7-pound, 3-ounce Viva was swimming in her newborn gown and cap, too—and wore 0-to-3-month onesies into her seventh month.

Onesies. The summer baby's rompers, these legless one-pieces with snaps at the crotch and long sleeves, short sleeves, or no sleeves are prime baby-wear once the umbilical stump has healed. You can make do with four, but if you're like me you probably received dozens during your shower. Avoid onesies with Velcro; they wreak havoc in the wash.

> "Don't worry if you don't know the art of swaddling, birthing experts will teach you."

Receiving blankets. The nurse who taught the birthing class I attended strongly recommended we pocket a few of the flannel baby blankets at the hospital. While I'm not saying you should pilfer anything, I am telling you that there is no better blanket for swaddling Baby, period. If you ask the nurses, they will probably give you permission to take a few. Many menagerie members are also fans of the Amazing Miracle Swaddle Blanket or the standard stretchy waffle-weave blanket. Whatever the case, four blankets should be enough. Even if your child hates being burrito-wrapped, you'll find lots of uses for them. By the way, don't worry if you don't know the art of swaddling; hospital nurses or other birthing experts will teach you.

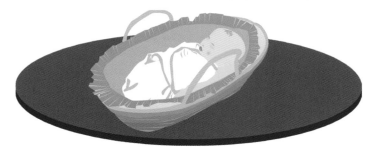

Rompers. Long or short sleeved, long legged, and with or without feet, these pajama-like one-pieces are VERY useful. Start with six and skip anything with buttons. Clothing with snaps is your new best friend.

Sleep sacks. New baby sleep sacks are essentially nightgowns that zip or snap at the bottom to create an instant sleeping bag. Get three.

Snowsuit and bunting. Whether you need them depends on where you live.

T-shirts and kimono-style shirts. Until the umbilical cord stump falls off (usually by three weeks), it's recommended that you avoid onesies, which are more constricting around the tummy. Instead, go for side-snap T-shirts or kimono-style shirts, which wrap and snap in the front so you don't have to pull anything over Baby's bobbling head. They're still no fun, as dressing a delicate and floppy new baby is a truly terrifying experience. Buy four just in case the hospital won't part with a few for free.

The Nursery

Whether you have a designated baby room or are sharing quarters, you will want a few furnishings and accoutrements to make your life easier.

A bed for Baby. Some people sleep with their newborns while others go straight to the crib, bassinette, cradle, Moses basket, or co-sleeper (a safe-snoozing appendage that attaches to the side of your bed). While not completely necessary, it is nice to use a tiny bed before you graduate to the crib. As one menagerie member said, "A crib seems way too big for them to sleep in right away." If you go the transitional bed route, I highly recommend you get something that can easily be moved from room to room. I had a hand-me-down bassinette on wheels, which was great for moving our sleeping girl around the house with us. If you buy a crib, build the cost of a mattress, which is sold separately, into your budget. Look for one that is fairly hard and snugly fits your crib.

Bedding. Whether you want a fancy bumper and matching everything is up to you. However, take note that bumpers are currently discouraged by the medical industry in fear of their possible contribution to Sudden Infant Death Syndrome (SIDS). What you do need, regardless of whether you have a bassinette, crib, or other, are at least three snug fitted sheets. You'll be amazed at how messy a tiny being can be.

If your crib linen comes with a blanket, tuck it away for the long haul; loose bedding is considered a SIDS risk. A far better choice for keeping Baby warm is a sleep sack (see above). A good thick gown or pajamas can also keep Baby cozy.

Changing table. This fancy piece of nursery furniture is nothing more than a tall table or low dresser with a strapped-on contoured pad and shelf or drawer space for all of the necessary accoutrements. It's awfully handy, but you can also make do by strapping on a contoured pad to a dresser or, if you're a serious minimalist, change your tot on the bed or the floor (although leaning that low can be the straw that breaks the new mommy's

Sensitive Soap Tip

The soap you use to wash your baby's clothes is just as important as attire itself. Buy gentle, hypoallergenic varieties designed specifically for baby's soft skin. They are available at all grocers. Buy a case to start because you will soon be doing laundry like it's your job.

aching back). The table or dresser is usually high enough that it's not so hard on you, plus the options for an older baby to turn over and escape without a diaper are much more limited. Personally, I found buying a proper table worth the expense. Whatever you do, set your table up so there's wall space on either side to help left- and right-handers on diaper duty get good leverage, and make sure there's countertop space within arm's reach because you will need it.

Contoured table pad. If you are as paranoid as I was that my completely immobile newborn might magically flip off of the table before my very eyes (despite my hands and full body block), you will find solace in this pad. It dips in the middle like a little comfy nest, and fastens around the tabletop for security. That said, you must always keep one hand and one eye on your baby. My changing table came with a flat pad and I was really glad I swapped it out.

Glider or rocking chair. Not absolutely necessary but highly recommended, the glider rocks, literally and figuratively. Recent studies show that rocking a baby helps develop the brain (something to do with the inner ear), while recent bedtime routines prove it's also a heck of a lot of fun to snuggle up just you two and read "Goodnight Moon" for the millionth time. You can probably find a good used rocker or glider on craigslist.com or through a local mother's club, but if you buy new you can just as easily sell it at two-thirds of the retail price once you're finished with it.

Hamper. You've got to stash the never-ending mound of dirty clothes somewhere.

Mobile. It's not critical, but a bouquet of dangling images does give Baby something to look at, which is said to help brain development. Thing is, they become obsolete the minute your tot can reach for it. If you're looking to cut corners, you can just as easily draw some big black and red block images on white paper and tape them to the wall behind Baby's changing table or bassinette. Or do both, like we did.

Monitor. This must-have allows you to keep track of your tot while he or she is in another room. Some are sound-only, while fancier versions include video. Video functionality is a serious expense, but many mommies say it's worth a splurge if you can swing it. I didn't, but now that my daughter is 19 months and throwing bedtime fits I really wish I could see what she's up to without having to enter her room and elevate the tantrum. Still, you can easily get by with a sound-only monitor. I like the type that has two receivers—one for the bedroom and one for the living room—and is portable, provided you've got fresh batteries.

Pad covers. Buy at least two so that you're prepared for the gazillion times Baby springs a surprise leak halfway through a change.

Feeding Essentials

Regardless of whether you're breastfeeding or formula feeding, you'll need the following items.

Bottle Sterilizer. Of course you can sterilize your bottles in boiling water. But a good backup plan is this steaming bag, which sterilizes bottles and nipples in three minutes flat when popped in the microwave with a few ounces of water. No, it's not PC, but it was the best alternative for me when traveling; sometimes it's a lot easier to track down a microwave than a stovetop, pot, and water.

> **Be Breast Prepared**
> Buy a book on breast-feeding. Seriously. See page 244 for specific recommendations. Also locate and note local resources in case you need them.

Bottle warmer. Minimalist that I am, I balked at the notion of buying this convenient contraption, but when a girlfriend gave me one it proved invaluable. It heats a bottle of milk or formula much faster than the alternatives—and that meant the world to me when listening to my tiny girl wail with hunger for even a few extra excruciating minutes.

Bottlebrush. If you've got bottles, you've got to clean 'em. These make cleaning easier.

Bottles and nipples. Lots of menagerie members rightly warned that even if you breastfeed it's wise to have a few bottles and nipples on hand in case you need to serve expressed milk or an emergency formula feeding. When scouting your options, be sure to buy a silicone nipple in the size intended for newborns. (Yes, there are nipple sizes; the larger the size, the faster the flow.) Also, if you are concerned about the chemicals in plastic bottles and want to know which brands are safer than others, search on "baby bottles" on The Green Guide (www.thegreenguide.com). Or just buy glass bottles, which are making a comeback. Whatever the case, four bottles is enough for starters.

Burp cloths. I laughed when I read what Brigette wrote about these: "Bought 'em. Never used 'em. I always forgot." I couldn't have said it better myself. I did buy a batch of cloth diapers with the intention of using them as burp cloths—and they definitely would have been better targets for the spit-up and other fun stuff I often ended up wearing. But ultimately, I never had a burp cloth in hand at the optimal time and ended up lining the bassinette with them so that when Viva spit up I could remove and replace the cloth without changing the bed sheet. I still have three gorgeous unused burp cloths in the bottom of Viva's dresser.

Formula. You may plan to use formula right out of the womb or end up needing to supplement your own supply.

The Mommy Menagerie On ...Did you have a vaginal birth or C-section?

97 mommies, who collectively gave birth 102 times, recalled their delivery room experiences and served up these stats, which suggest the amount of major abdominal surgeries known as C-sections are on the rise, whether elected or prescribed.

Vaginal Births	59%
C-Sections	41%

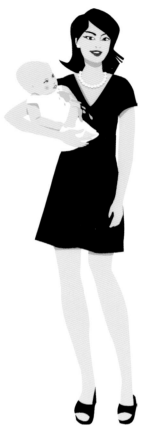

Regardless, there are enough formula pushers in the medical community that you've probably already received a few free cans. Keep 'em. You'll never know if and when you might need them and the stuff is expensive! If you're buying for the long haul, check out supersize portions at discount food outlets like Costco or 1800diapers.com.

Nursing pillow. An absolutely critical purchase, this wrap-around-the-waist pillow will stop you from slumping forward and ruining your back every time your tot wants a breast or bottle. Bring it to the hospital and use it from the first feeding on. Most mommies I know prefer the Boppy pillow. I didn't think My Breast Friend was all that chummy, despite it's name, because the Velcro waistband scared the bejeezus out of sleeping Viva when I'd try to take it off.

Breastfeeding

Believe it or not, you need lots of expensive gizmos, even if you're going the mother's milk route.

Breast-milk storage bags. Even if you're committed to busting out a boob on demand until your kid goes to college, it's still smart to pump and refrigerate or freeze some breast milk in specially made bags. You'll reach for them if you have to take medication you don't want your baby to ingest, want to drink a few glasses of wine without passing the buzz to Baby (in which case you give stored milk and "pump and dump" your wine-tainted milk), or find yourself low in internal supply for some reason.

Breast pads. I never used these, but many mommies do.

Breast pump. If you're breastfeeding, you'll want one of these. You can rent one from a hospital, but if you're anteing up for a purchase, go with "Medela Pump in Style." It's a double-barrel electric model with a coy carrying case and a battery pack for pumping on the go.

Believe it or not, I regularly used mine while driving to and from my job. Despite the likelihood of being busted by truckers in their tall cabs, it was when I was the most relaxed, which is essential for good results. Had I been pulled over, my calmness surely would have been spoiled. But in that case, I would definitely have milked my embarrassment for all it was worth.

Forget manual pumps. You're not a cow on the farm.

Nipple cream. Nursing can be a sore spot for most mommies—especially in the beginning. Ease the pain of overused, cracked, and bleeding nipples with any brand of this special baby-friendly lotion. Lots of mommies like Lansinoh or Aquaphor, which also works wonders on diaper rash.

Bathing

Baby won't be ready for the tub for a while. But he will need his own toiletries.

Baby wash. Newborns don't have much opportunity to get grit under their nails or behind their ears, so you don't need more than a mild all-in-one hair and body wash—and you shouldn't even use that for the first few weeks. I seek out organic stuff that is mild on the skin, eyes, and offensive ingredients.

Bathtub. For me the only thing more intimidating than clipping my newborn's nails were her first few baby baths. A contoured tub, which props the baby up for you, made it easier on all of us. It's good for the sponge-bath stage, while you're waiting for Baby's umbilical stump to jump ship, and beyond—so long as you never ever leave your little one unattended anywhere near water.

Towels. As much as you probably want me to tell you that the adorable hooded towels are essential, alas they are not. Any soft fluffy towel will do when drying your new baby. But that doesn't mean you shouldn't buy a few anyway. They will last long after your kid gets that wearing his towel makes him look like a dinosaur.

Washcloths. You may as well buy a pack of washcloths made just for Baby, because it'll cost about as much as one good-quality, grown-up cloth elsewhere. A nice sponge works just as well. Whatever you buy, anticipate that it will do double-duty because as soon as he is able, Baby will insist on sucking on it.

The Mommy Menagerie On ...Who Delivered Their Babies

I had no idea how likely it was that someone other than my appointed OB-GYN would help me welcome my girl into the world. Turns out, substitutes are actually somewhat common, as is indicated by percentages below, which pertain to a total of 90 births.

Delivery Director	% of Moms Who They Helped
Primary Doctor	63%
Substitute or Partner in Practice	32%
Midwife	2%
Other	4%

"Buy in advance to avoid racing to the drugstore in the middle of the night."

Baby Care

Don't forget any of these health- and beauty-related buys.

Comb and brush. I bought these a month before Viva was born and 20 months later they still haven't been used. Most babies don't have enough hair to comb, but at some point they will. In the meantime, they look cute on the dresser.

Cotton swabs. Only for use with the alcohol mentioned on page 221, cotton swabs have no place on any other portion of a babe's body, period.

Humidifier/vaporizer. You probably won't need this contraption that helps clear a baby's stuffy nose until you really need it (like at midnight when your kid is throwing a fit because he can't sleep without being able to breathe through his nostrils). Then you will wish you already owned it. Skip other brands and go straight to the model made by Vicks.

Infant gas drops. You might want to start with the natural gas reliever known as "gripe water" for easing Baby's bubbly tummy, but if she doesn't like it or it doesn't work you'll quickly and gladly graduate to the bright pink, over-the-counter Infants' Mylicon. Whatever you choose, get an extra bottle. Trust me: You do not want to find yourself in need and without.

Infants' Tylenol. You won't need this right out of the womb, but the first time your pediatrician recommends you use it, you will wish you already had it. Better to buy in advance than to race to the drugstore in the middle of the night toting a bawling and feverish babe. FYI: Don't dose your baby without specific direction from your pediatrician.

Nail clippers. For me, clipping nails on tiny newborn fingers was one of the most horrifying jobs of new motherhood. There's so much margin for error, yet it's a must since Baby's nails can go from manicured to Freddy Krueger-like in less than a week. Best bet is to ease into it by first filing nails with a baby emery board, buying a few clippers, and discovering which is most comfortable for you. I found the supermini Swiss Army knife, recommended by my birthing-class instructor and available at places like Target, was easiest and safest to maneuver. Brigette prefers the Safety First or Gerber miniature toenail clippers.

The Truth about Birthing
What does it feel like to give birth? It's every mother's burning question. More than one mommy has offered an answer that isn't particularly pretty or comprehensible unless you've been there: Plainly put, giving birth feels like shitting a watermelon—seriously.

Nasal aspirator. Your hospital or birthing center should give you a parting gift of one of these bulbous, baster-like booger-suckers. But you should still get a few extras. They're great for clearing Baby's clogged nostrils or even grabbing spit-up or other goo that hasn't made its way out of the mouth. I kept one in the diaper bag and one stuck in the corner of the bassinette for the first few months, and was happy to still have a backup when one split at its seam.

Petroleum jelly. This slippery stuff is very helpful during those first weeks when applying it to Baby's bottom will help make the tar-like newborn poo easier to wipe off, and slathering it over circumcision incisions will help with healing. It can later be used to help ease in a rectal thermometer, and to keep the skin beneath a runny nose moist.

Rubbing alcohol. Keep a small bottle at your changing table and use it to gently clean your baby's umbilical stump, unless your doctor advises otherwise; my editor's doc told her to simply keep the stump dry.

Thermometer. Get a digital one that can be used in three places (oral, rectal, under the arm).

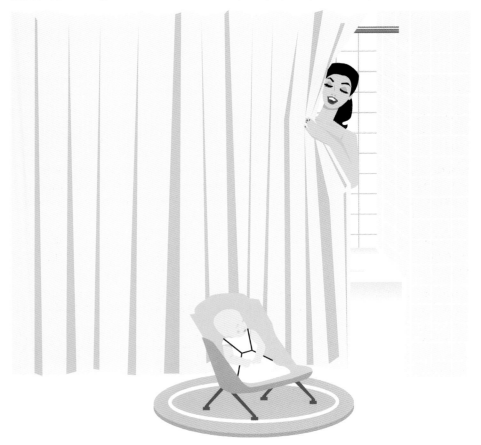

Baby Gear

There is a dizzying array of goods designed to help your baby be more easily transported. My advice when you face the tidal wave of options is start with the basics. Once you have your child you'll have a better idea about what else you might need or want.

Car window shade. Block direct sun on both back seat windows with cheap and easy-to-apply shades, or your baby will squint and complain when in transit.

Pack 'n Play. These baby boxing rings are not a necessity, but certainly a convenience for the first year. Some brands include bassinette functionality (a snap-on sheet that makes the surface higher) so you can use it as a makeshift changing table or a satellite napping station. They also double as a toy corral and portable bed for overnight trips. However, some babies won't stand for them.

> "Start with the basics. Once you have your child you'll have a better idea of what you need."

Rear-facing infant car seat or infant-toddler (aka convertible) car seat. Gotta have it. Brigette gave the Graco SnugRide props. I was happy with a Peg Perego model, which I inherited. Both have a seat that snaps into a base installed into your car, which is a huge plus because you can carry the seat—with Baby in it—everywhere you go. (Essential for grocery store runs, transporting a sleeping baby from the car to the house, or even as an ad hoc bed for babies with reflux.) If you have two people driving Miss Baby, you only need an extra base—the car seat can interchange with either of them. You'll need to trade up once the baby is 20 pounds, however.

If you get a convertible style car seat, you don't need to buy a bigger seat as quickly because they can carry tots up to 65 pounds. But you lose the convenience of carrying that infant seat around. Plus, if you are using two cars, you will probably want two of them, as you can't easily change it out. Whatever you get, practice using it BEFORE you put a baby in it. I tried to adjust the tightness of ours for the first time with our newborn strapped into it and nearly strangled her. It was not a comforting and confidence-boosting induction into motherhood.

Sling/soft carrier. It's your call on this one. Some moms swear by them because they allow for hands-free tot toting and allow Baby to be next to your heart at all times. I didn't warm up to them or the Baby Bjorn, which we bought but probably used a whopping three times.

Stroller. Unless you have nowhere to go, you do need one of these. I'm cuckoo for the Graco travel system, because you can snap its aforementioned infant car seat into a coordinating stroller while the baby is still less than

20 pounds. This functionality is especially handy when your baby is too small and young to sit up on his or her own. Once your child is a little older, the stroller can be used without the snap-in seat for a few years.

Baby Fun & Comfort

Fun and comfort don't benefit merely your Mini Me. You'll soon see that there's little you won't do to soothe your unsettled little one or bring a toothless smile to his pudgy little face. These are some items that may help you make jovial or tranquil magic for your entire family.

Batteries. Once you learn how many batteries it takes to keep Baby marveling at the mobile and bopping in the bouncy seat, you'll wish you invested in Eveready. Inventory all of the sizes your gizmos take and buy three times what you think you need.

Bouncy seat. If you can only splurge on one item, this should be it. Versions with vibrating, musical, and visual elements are virtual newborn-sitters that will keep your kid preoccupied or coax her to pass out long enough for you to actually do something for yourself—like eat, change your underwear, or shower (with one eye on the babe, of course). My girl was ga-ga for Fisher Price's Ocean Wonders seat, while Brigette preferred the quieter Kick & Play.

Gym or play mat. Long before I was a mom, I regularly gave a fancy play mat with fun things dangling overhead as a baby shower gift (my favorite is Tiny Love Super Deluxe Gymini with Lights and Music). But it was only when I had reason to own one myself that I understood why they're so wonderful. These colorful quilts give Baby lots to look at long before she can scoot around and grab the dangling toys, lick the plastic mirror, and marvel at the flashing lights. They also fold up easily, can be set up anywhere, and provide a clean spot for some back or tummy time on any floor.

Pacifier. You probably have your own position on pacifiers, so I'm not going to preach about their perks and pitfalls. All I'll say is that if you decide to partake, buy silicone suckers, which are rumored to be safer in the carcinogen-releasing department than latex or rubber counterparts.

Stroller, crib, and car-seat toys. They come as plush colorful animals or shapes and attach to a stroller, crib, or car seat via Velcro or hard plastic links. Get one or two.

"You'll soon see that there's little you won't do to soothe your unsettled little one."

The New Baby Starter Kit Checklist Cheat Sheet

Diapering
- ☐ Diapers (100+)
- ☐ Dry wipes (1 case)
- ☐ Wipes (1 case)
- ☐ Diaper bag
- ☐ Diaper pail or garbage can
- ☐ Diaper rash ointment

Clothing & Blankets
- ☐ T-shirts or kimono-style shirts (4)
- ☐ Gowns (3)
- ☐ Hats (2 to 3)
- ☐ Onesies (6)
- ☐ Rompers (4)
- ☐ Receiving or swaddle blankets (4)
- ☐ Sleep sacks (2 to 3)
- ☐ Booties or socks (none or 1 pack)
- ☐ Snowsuit and bunting (if you need it)
- ☐ Laundry detergent (1 case)

The Nursery
- ☐ Changing table
- ☐ Contoured table pad
- ☐ Pad covers (2)
- ☐ A bed and mattress for baby
- ☐ Fitted sheets (3)
- ☐ Monitor
- ☐ Glider or rocking chair
- ☐ Hamper
- ☐ Mobile (optional)

Feeding Essentials
- ☐ Bottles and nipples (4)
- ☐ Bottlebrush (2)
- ☐ Nursing pillow
- ☐ Formula
- ☐ Bottle sterilizer
- ☐ Bottle warmer
- ☐ Burp cloths

Breastfeeding
- ☐ Breast pump
- ☐ Breast-milk storage bags
- ☐ Breast pads
- ☐ Nipple cream

Bathing
- ☐ Bathtub
- ☐ Baby wash
- ☐ Towels
- ☐ Washcloths

Baby Care
- ☐ Nasal aspirator (2)
- ☐ Comb and brush
- ☐ Infant gas drops (2)
- ☐ Infant Tylenol (2)
- ☐ Teething tablets or gel
- ☐ Nail clippers or files
- ☐ Thermometer
- ☐ Humidifier/vaporizer
- ☐ Petroleum jelly
- ☐ Rubbing alcohol (optional)
- ☐ Cotton swabs (optional)

Baby Gear
- ☐ Rear-facing infant car seat or infant-toddler (aka convertible) car seat
- ☐ Car window shades
- ☐ Pack 'n Play (optional)
- ☐ Sling/soft carrier (optional)
- ☐ Stroller

Baby Fun & Comfort (optional)
- ☐ Pacifier
- ☐ Bouncy seat
- ☐ Stroller, crib, and car-seat toys
- ☐ Swing
- ☐ Gym or play mat
- ☐ Batteries

For You and Your Sanity
- ☐ Maxi-pads
- ☐ Car infant mirror
- ☐ Parenting book

Swing. Babies either love or hate the swing. But parents that have swinger babies are beyond stoked, because when the bouncy seat loses its luster, these battery-operated swaying contraptions can rock the fussiest baby into a tranquil bundle of sleeping joy. They plummet in popularity the minute your munchkin can maneuver, but in the midst of the earliest months most parents will do anything for some respite. Brigette and I are fans of Fisher Price's Aquarium Ocean Wonders Cradle Swing. It ain't cheap, but you can easily resell it for at least 50% of the price. Buy it from a local source so if your baby rejects it right out of the box, you can easily return it.

A Few More Items For You

Grab these random goods, which aid in your mental and physical transitions.

Car infant mirror. If you can't bear the idea of driving around without being able to confirm that your baby is alive and well at any given moment, a front-view mirror is your savior. Securely placed and properly angled, it allows you and your baby to ogle each other despite a rear-facing car seat.

Maxi pads. Whether you have a vaginal birth or a C-section, you will still bleed for up to six weeks after your baby is born. Load up on a couple of boxes of maxi pads; tampons are recovery no-nos.

A parenting book. Even if you buy a book that tells you everything you need to know about being a new mom and caring for a newborn, you may still call the pediatrician and your mommy girlfriends nineteen times in the first few weeks. Still, a good manual may stop you from calling your best friend yet again because you need baby-burping pointers. For a recommendation, see "Sources" on page 243.

I want to share something with you that I didn't hear enough about before I had my baby: The first six months are really hard. Women who were born to be mommies will disagree, but those of us who have enjoyed being self-indulgent rulers of our own domains and defined ourselves through professional or social accomplishments might beg to differ. Yes, listening to sweet coos, tickling tiny toes, and cuddling a newborn is enough to regularly make your heart feel fuller than your new-mommy breasts. In fact, if you're like me, you might find yourself regularly overwhelmed with emotion, blubbering uncontrollably at the most mundane thing, like singing "Twinkle, Twinkle, Little Star" to your four-week-old.

But in conjunction with moments of parental glory is the relentless and all-consuming task of navigating new parenthood, caring for a newborn, and realizing that you and your desires are no longer the first priorities in your own life. This is when brushing your teeth or taking a shower becomes a luxury and you may cry just as much out of joy as out of exhaustion, fear, frustration, and the horror that you will be nothing more than a slave to a completely needy being for the rest of your days.

Before you panic and wonder whether you can trade in your tot for something more freewheeling like a red convertible sports car, let me tell you the thing that you will soon hear over and over again because it is true: It gets better.

You are about to enter one of life's most dramatic transitions. It does change you and your life forever, and it comes with never-ending challenges. But trust me when I say that the benefits far outweigh the struggles, even for someone like me who couldn't see that there was actually a light at the end of the new motherhood tunnel until I got there—and that was a solid six months after Viva was born.

Here's my advice to any mother who finds herself loving her child but having a hard time embracing her new life, running on no sleep, or staying in sync with her partner: Remember that this experience really is fleeting. Right now your baby is the most helpless and least reciprocal: You give, give, and give, and your little blob takes, takes, and takes. The emotional drain is indescribable. But before you know it, your little one will be more self-sufficient and will sleep through the night. You will not call the doctor 20 times at the first sign of a stuffy nose or believe that life as you know it has come to an end. You will get into a rhythm, find ways to celebrate the old you from time to time, and get more joy out of the new person in your life than you could have imagined. To top it off, 18 months from now you won't remember anything about this time, which has got to be nature's way of encouraging you to add yet another younger to your brood.

WELCOME TO THE CLUB!

Congratulations! You made it! You've officially joined the ranks of the mommy menagerie. (Or maybe you're reading this chapter before the big day, which isn't a bad idea since new parents have little time to read.) I've kept this section short and sweet because there really isn't much to caring for a newborn other than to repeatedly feed, burp, diaper, cuddle, and soothe him or her. Besides, the minute I had my daughter I dropped the pregnancy books and picked up the baby-care tomes. I imagine you'll do the same. So, brush up on the need-to-know details and get on with enjoying that wrinkly ball of deliciousness, squeezing in naps, or arguing with your partner because you're too damned tired to do anything else.

RECOVERY ESSENTIALS

In order to take care of anyone else you must take care of yourself first—even if you aren't your first priority anymore. Your energy, attitude, and health—and thus your ability to care for your child—depend on it. So check out the following tips on how to heal and prosper as you navigate the wild and wacky world of motherhood.

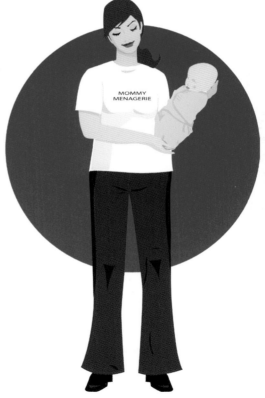

Monitor your bleeding.

You should have something similar to a heavy period for several days after giving birth vaginally or via C-section. If you are soaking more than one pad per hour or see big blood clots, call your provider ASAP.

Tend to your wounds.

If you had an episiotomy or tore during the birth, keep an eye on your perineum to make sure it doesn't get infected. Also keep the area clean and spray it with a spray bottle of warm water after going to the bathroom. If you had a C-section, check the incision area for infections. If it looks red or puffy or smells funky, call your provider pronto.

Watch for warning signs.

While most mommies don't have any serious postpartum problems, there are a few instances beyond those mentioned above in which you should call your provider immediately, specifically if you have a fever over 100.4°F or 38°C; intense abdominal pain; extremely painful, red, hot, or hard areas of the breast or calf; perpetual headaches; spots in front of your eyes; or depression.

Eat healthy food—regularly.

To keep your energy up you need all the help you can get right now. Make sure you take time to chow down, ideally on foods that are as comforting for your body as they are for your mind (i.e. preempt the chocolate ice cream with some chicken-broccoli stir fry).

Be nice to your nipples.

Wash them with warm water only—skip fancy soaps or moisturizers other than provider-approved nipple creams. If they are cracked during the first days, squeeze out and rub colostrum onto them, let them air dry as much as possible, and use a baby-safe lanolin cream.

Take naps.

I foolishly didn't follow this tip, but would have been much better off if I had. Sleep when the baby sleeps. A well-rested mommy is a saner parent and partner.

Hang back on sex until you're ready.

There is no rule of thumb on when to get back in the saddle. The right time to start depends on your physical and mental condition. Personally, I couldn't even think about doing the deed for a solid three months—and I had a C-section! Even then lubrication was in order because my yoo-hoo had been through such a hormonal ordeal.

Be patient.

Don't be surprised if it takes several weeks or even a couple of months for you to completely recover from giving birth. I have a couple of friends who delivered vaginally and waltzed around immediately afterward, but most mommies I know took at least a month to heal from vaginal or C-section births. The reason you don't hear more about this is because these recovering women are holed up dealing with newborns, an experience that trumps virtually everything else.

BABY CARE BASICS

Like I said before, there really isn't much to caring for a newborn. That will change soon enough, but for now you can subsist on this short-list of must-dos. It might not seem like much, but it will take all of your time.

Feed Baby on demand!

See "Feeding Facts" on page 231 for details.

Be diligent with diaper duty.

You will probably receive a sheet of paper from the hospital or birthing center that will tell you your tot should have about as many wet diapers as she is days old (i.e. three days old equals three wet diapers within 24 hours) and that his or her poop should change from black to yellow by the fifth day. If this isn't happening, or your baby doesn't have any wet diapers within 24 hours, call your pediatrician ASAP.

Mind the umbilical cord.

Baby's uterine feeding tube will slowly make its exit. Until then, keep it clean, occasionally gently brushing it with alcohol on a cotton swab, and call the pediatrician if the area becomes red, drains any type of liquid, or has a funky odor.

Get to know Baby's cries.

Although hearing your baby cry can be as uncomfortable as listening to a symphony of nails on a chalkboard, try to remember that it is your cutie pie's only way of communicating with you (until around a year from now when the word "No" becomes the expression of choice). Listen closely and soon you will be able to recognize whether a wail means, "I want food!" "Change my diaper!" or "Hold me, Mommy!"

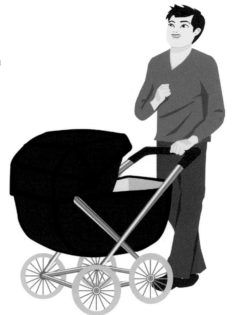

Comfort Baby.

Other than a full tummy, a dry diaper, good burping, and a cozy outfit, comfort is the best way to ease a fussy baby. It can come in myriad forms, including you or your partner walking the baby (something my husband did for at least an hour early each morning for the first weeks), rocking, laying her against your chest (ideally bare), letting Baby suckle on a nipple, finger, or pacifier, using a vibrating bouncy seat or white noise, swaddling, or administering baby-safe, gas-relief medicine (gas is new parents' greatest foe). Try various tricks, see what works, and stick with it until invariably Baby changes his mind and wants something new. Then try everything all over again.

Position Baby for safe sleep.

All the pros say positioning Baby on his or her back is a preventative measure against SIDS, as is keeping the crib or bassinette clear of blankets, pillows, and stuffed animals for at least the first year (my girl is nearly two and still does just fine with nothing but a mattress with a sheet, bumper, a sleep sack, and her teddy bear "Bop").

Taking Your Tot's Temperature
A normal temperature for Baby is 97.6°F to 98.9°F (36.5°C to 37.5°C). If you think your baby has a fever, take her temperature under her arm and call the pediatrician immediately if you are right.

Check for jaundice.

After three days you should take a peek at Baby's bare body and make sure it's a nice healthy pink. If your little one has a yellow hue, or a yellowing of the whites of his eyes, contact your pediatrician ASAP for easy but important remedies.

Keep Baby comfy.

If he's too hot or too cold he may cry to clue you in. Regardless, the rule of thumb is to dress or wrap Baby in one more layer than you would wear.

Bathe Baby.

New babies don't play hard enough to work up a sweat or to get dirt under their nails, so they really don't need to be bathed all that often. A sponge bath once a week with nothing but warm water and a soft facecloth should do it—and don't forget to keep Baby's body out of water until his umbilical stump has abandoned ship.

Make a pediatric appointment.

You should tote your tot to the doctor's office for a well visit according to your pediatrician's instructions. Often a visit is scheduled the first week after birth, and then again one or two weeks later. Once you get home and settled, call to schedule a date.

Baby 911 Cheat Sheet

Call the pediatrician immediately if Baby . . .

❑ Still has black stools on the fifth day or has more than six to eight watery stools a day.

❑ Refuses to eat and has missed two feedings.

❑ Has not had a wet diaper in 24 hours.

❑ Is listless, lethargic, restless, or irritable, or becomes "floppy" and loses muscle tone.

❑ Has a fever.

❑ Is wheezing, congested, or has flaring nostrils or trouble breathing.

❑ Has a swollen, stinky, or oozing umbilical cord.

❑ Is yellow (jaundiced).

❑ Projectile vomits or spits-up frequently.

❑ Had a circumcision that is swollen or bleeding.

FEEDING FACTS

A baby's first few weeks are all about mealtimes. Luckily, he's not yet ready to demand quesadillas or chicken nuggets. Gobble up the following feeding facts and you'll be prepared to help that little bean grow big and strong.

Feed Baby whenever he or she is hungry.

You should expect your little one to politely lick his or her lips, root around, or more blatantly bellow that it's snack time every one and a half to three hours, and more frequently as he hits growth spurts down the road. Oblige him or her with the boob or a bottle, but make sure it happens at least eight times within each 24-hour period. (Keeping a written record helps sleepless parents who find the day becomes one blurry mess of diapers and milk.) If Baby is a heavy enough sleeper to snooze through mealtime, gently wake him for a feeding until your pediatrician advises otherwise. Good nutrition now will help everyone relax later.

If you're breastfeeding...

Your milk won't come in for about three days. Those first days feed Baby on demand, but limit nursing to 15 minutes per breast per feeding so he gets as much colostrom (nutrient-rich pre-milk) as possible.

Once your milk comes in, Baby should suckle at least every one to three hours for 15 to 30 minutes on one breast before you burp him and move to boob number two for a second course. If Baby forgoes the option, express or pump the milk from that breast and start your wee one on the full breast next go-round. Then try shortening the time to 10 to 15 minutes on each side, always starting on the side you finished with. (A good way to remember which boob is up to bat is to keep a rubber band around your wrist and alternate it from your left to right arm to indicate which side to start on next time.)

Do not skip your baby's feedings to catch up on sleep. Be sure to eat enough—at least an extra 500 calories per day—and stay hydrated; slacking off on any of these can deplete your milk supply.

Babies get "milk drunk" and can doze off halfway through a feeding. Keep her perky by tickling the side of her face or the bottom of her feet.

> ### Try to Be Open-Minded
>
> If you intend to breastfeed, go into it with the right mind-set. Breastfeeding is recommended for optimum infant health, but as one menagerie member pointed out, though it is natural, it does not always come naturally to women and there is no one right way to do it. She warned, "I felt like with all the breastfeeding books out there, the comments from organizations like Le Leche League, and even in the breast-feeding classes everything seems so black and white, like it's all or nothing. I think this scares the crap out of women and sets them up for failure."

If you're having latching or other problems, do not hesitate to contact a lactation consultant or your practitioner to learn of ways to work it out.

Don't take any medications without consulting with your practitioners, as they can transfer to breast milk.

If you're bottle-feeding

Baby should have two to four ounces of formula (never cow's milk or anything else that has not been approved by your childcare provider) every two to four hours. Burp that ball of joy after every ½ to 1 ounce.

ADJUSTING TO YOUR NEW LIFE

Even if you've been dreaming of being a mother since you were a little girl, you may still find the transition to parenthood challenging, frightening, and exhausting. If this is true for you, read on for empathy and tips on how to make sure you aren't brought to tears as often as your newborn.

Don't expect too much

too soon. Parenting requires stamina that is built up over time. It's like running a marathon: With training you can plug along at an even keel and hardly break a sweat, but those first few months of practice can leave the novice on the verge of collapse. (This is especially important to remember if you are your child's primary caretaker and your partner pitches in on weekends. Watch and see how quickly he or she wilts without continuous practice—then try to be sympathetic rather than wanting to kill him or her because they should be grateful that you're doing the lion's share.) Don't be surprised if it takes you a while to get comfortable with your new role. Instead remind yourself that you're going through an adjustment period, that all new skills take time to master, and soon your parenthood will be second nature.

"Embrace any fears as evidence that you are a caring, protective mother, talk about them with someone who can relate, and let them pass."

Make time to regroup.

Motherhood is exhausting stuff. Preemptively stealing moments to replenish your soul, energy, and spirit goes a long way, even if it's by doing something as simple as taking a walk around the block or dashing out for a quick pedicure. But it's especially important if you find yourself losing your patience, cool, or mind. The last thing you want to do is take it out on Baby. (Reminder: NEVER shake a baby; results can include brain damage and fatality.) Your partner, on the other hand, is likely to have to lump it. Give yourself some space to reinvigorate and, by the time your baby says, "Hi Mommy!" in a singsong voice guaranteed to make your heart melt even when it's 2:30 in the morning, you will be emotionally available enough to truly savor it.

Know that fear is natural.

First the bad news: Now that you have this cherished being in your care, you will always have something to worry about. The thought of SIDS may have you sleeping with one eye open. Later, a nasty flu, fearlessness on the jungle gym, and—heaven help us—dating and high school peer pressure will probably have us all biting our nails down to nubs. But the good news is that if you are experiencing as much fear as you are elation around your baby's well being, you will definitely become less paranoid as time passes. The first six months I obsessed about SIDS, Viva choking on her spit-up, and the random possibility of someone breaking into the house and kidnapping our daughter in the middle of the night. We all survived it. Embrace any fears as evidence that you are a caring, protective mother, talk about them with someone who can relate, and let them pass.

Instant Glamour

Though it's not essential, one of the things that perked me up during the early days of motherhood was a stash of instant glamour products. These were beauty items and accessories that took seconds to apply but magically made me feel a little pampered and pretty when I hardly had time to brush my hair. My favorites were a variety of lip glosses, Kiehl's Creme With Silk Groom hairstyling cream, a few fancy headbands, and Benefit Cosmetics Speed Brow because it pronounced my eyebrows and distracted me from the bags under my eyes. Find a few fast saviors, take a moment to preen, and you may feel better about yourself—even if your baby is the only person who sees you all day.

Air out any frustrations.

I believe discussions about the frustrations of motherhood are often only shared in whispers among close friends because many mothers are afraid of being judged, or fear that voicing their complaints makes them sound as if they don't love their children. My thought on that is: Get over it. After I had my baby and was having trouble adjusting to a life of servitude in conjunction with a new marriage, a new home, a new community, and the loss of my personal identity, I happily broke the motherhood code of silence. When people asked me how it was going, I often said, "Having a daughter rocks, but being a mother sucks." While some people (other than mommies) were surprised to hear it, I didn't care. I believe a realistic

Life as You'll Never Know It

Here's a parental truism you will soon know all to well: As a parent you'll experience life as a series of the longest days and the shortest years.

Mommy Menagerie On ...How would you sum up pregnancy as an experience?

As you can now attest, capturing the wild world of pregnancy in words is no easy task, but the menagerie gave it a good shot. Here are some highlights.

"An incredibly transformative experience in a very short time."

"For me it was wonderful and completely freaky all at once."

"A test. It changes everything about you so that you can embrace the new side of yourself: a mother."

"Pregnancy is a journey of wonderment and ecstasy. It brings the five senses to its highest potential and perhaps allows one to discover one's sixth sense—intuition."

"I thought it was magical. I loved that my female body was doing what needed to be done all on its own and that there was this person growing within me. I felt very important and special—even though everywhere I turned there were other pregnant women. "

"Full of uncertainties and truly a miracle–we get very few opportunities to participate in a miracle."

"It takes forever and goes by all too quickly."

"Pregnancy is an amazing journey that brings a woman many conflicting experiences from sickness to satisfaction, from pain to comfort and, in the end, the most joy one could ever imagine."

"It's an emotional rollercoaster inside your body. People can actually see you physically going up, but they can't see you going emotionally up and down. You will return to being alone at the end, you will be changed for the experience, and for sure you feel quite woozy after the ride."

"Wild and necessary. One big science experiment that brings a couple closer."

"Like you are merely a host for an insane science experiment going on in your body."

"For me pregnancy's been an exciting and obsessive-compulsive experience. It has made me realize how strong, healthy, and totally vulnerable I am."

"It was a real roller coaster. I was shocked I was pregnant and with my depression struggled a great deal initially. Once I was under better care and took care of my health issues I was able to enjoy the tail end of the experience. And it's important to know that less than 12 hrs after I had my son, I told my husband I wanted another child! Whatever we suffer, the end result is worth it!"

"It's the most universally respected, admired, supported, awe-inspiring, and thrilling experience I've ever known."

"The most amazing thing that we are lucky enough to get to experience. I feel sorry for men!"

"Magical! It's easy to get wrapped up in all of the discomfort, inconvenience, and anticipation. But don't lose sight of what's actually happening: an actual life is being created--a tiny little person is growing and developing and becoming your baby!"

and honest perspective on parenting helps other new mommies prepare themselves and get through it in one happy, healthy piece.

If you are struggling with your transition, try joining a playgroup, talking to mommy friends, seeking professional help, visiting online chat rooms, or dropping me a line through my website, TheRealDealGuide.com. You'll quickly discover you're not alone.

> ### Get That Baby on Tape
>
> Take videos of your baby even if she doesn't seem to do anything other than eat and sleep. A year from now and forever after, you will look back in amazement and be glad that you caught those dreamy, otherwise forgotten, moments on tape.

Be flexible.

Sometimes having a newborn is like riding a roller coaster in the dark. You never know when the big dips, climbs, and turns are going to come. To make matters even more exhilarating, the minute you get into a rhythm and can anticipate the highs, lows, and in betweens, the routine changes. The best thing to do is enjoy the ride. That way you can find humor in the unexpected—like the time Colie, Viva, and I arrived 45 minutes late to our neighbor's house for a luncheon in our honor because on our way out the door the baby barfed on her first outfit, needed a diaper change once she was in her second ensemble, and then insisted on a third costume change by peeing halfway through the diaper swap. Speaking of, getting ready, leaving the house, and virtually everything else takes longer when you have a baby, so try to keep your schedule as flexible as possible.

Don't worry about your weight for at least a year.

You've got bigger shoes to fill now, so you may as well embrace the body that goes with them—especially if you are breastfeeding. Nursing moms are encouraged not to lose weight quickly, as it may jeopardize milk supply. Some women naturally look like they were never pregnant three months after the fact, but the rest of us need to give ourselves a break, focus on motherhood, and reassess down the road. Trust me when I tell you that if you make losing your extra weight a priority when the time comes, you will do it.

Make time for your partner.

Even the happiest couples will tell you that new parenthood brings out the beast in them. The best way to reconnect with your partner in the throes of this transition is to find a little time now and then for just the two of you. If that's not possible, batten down the hatches and wait out the storm. Then, if and when time

> ### Get Out of the House
>
> Once you get comfortable with caring for your baby, get out of the house and have some fun with your new family. Early on, babies are very portable and their schedules are flexible. This is a time when you can take them out to lunch as they snooze safely in their carriers, or even do as we did and check into a hotel and indulge in a two-hour dinner while our child slept next to the dining room table. Once your little one develops a sleep schedule, you'll be far more restricted and have to do what I call "running the nap gauntlet," which is essentially hanging out at home and making mad dashes to do errands between naptimes.

the storm. Then, if and when time and resources permit, schedule a regular date night. It'll do wonders for your relationship.

Remember that your partner is adjusting too.

You've been having a very close relationship with your little schmoo for the past three trimesters. But this is when reality—and the ability to participate—may really hit your partner. When the meconium (aka black-tar newborn poo) hits the fan, remind yourself that you're not the only one going through a major adjustment and be as sympathetic as your patience and energy level allow.

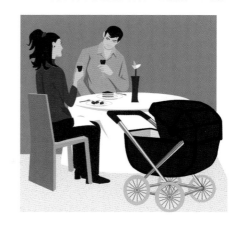

Roll with the punches as best you can.

There is no way to anticipate or orchestrate how this new time will go. So now that you're in the passenger seat, you may as well take advantage of it. Rather than try to backseat-drive, just go along for the ride. The view is truly spectacular if you take time to look.

ONE FINAL WORD

The most intriguing thing I've discovered about motherhood is that it bonds all of us together. Whenever I see a pregnant woman, think of someone reading this book while expecting, or learn that a friend is about to give birth, my heart literally bulges inside my chest, my eyes well up, and I feel deeply moved. It's not that I am an overly sensitive person. It's that the prospect of bringing a bright new spirit into the world and everything that comes afterward perpetually humbles me, and makes me feel deeply connected to those who undertake the often underrated and extremely generous act. All of our pregnancies, lives, and circumstances may be dramatically different but, in the end, we are all mothers and this common bond is stronger than any other I've experienced.

But motherhood has changed my perspective on more than just the women with children around me. Now that I am a mom, I literally look at everyone with a little more love in my heart because I know that each and every person is somebody's baby. For me it's a profoundly moving thought, which has made me a kinder, more considerate, and forgiving person. As painful as that sensitivity can be at times, I am happy for it.

As you move into this new, challenging, gratifying, and very tender role you will surely have your own experiences and revelations. I just want you to know that as a fellow mother my heart is truly with you and your family, and I wish you a lifetime of joy, wonderment, patience, and love. Congratulations, and don't forget to book yourself a massage!

Warmly,

Erika Lenkert

Books and Websites

Whether you're interested in obtaining one or more prenatal tomes, want some great Internet resources, or would like to read up on pregnancy particulars such as exercise, bed rest, or maneuvering while carrying multiples, you'll find a good selection of sources here. Also, check out my website, TheRealDealGuide.com, for updates, sympathy, and additional information.

General Reference Guides

What to Expect When You're Expecting
3rd Edition, by Heidi Murkoff, Arlene Eisenberg, and Sandee Hathaway, B.S.N., (Workman, 2002)

This encyclopedic, nonjudgmental, and heavily factual bible covers virtually every possible pregnancy circumstance. For better and worse, the spectrum includes the gamut of concerns and dilemmas, which can instill fear in even the healthiest, problem-free mommy-to-be. (One mommy I know called it "The Scary Book.") Still, it's good to grab if you have a question about any and everything. While I was pregnant, I kept one big fat book with all the gory details around for when I needed it. This was the one. One downside: Because it's organized by month, random details can be hard to find.

The Girlfriend's Guide to Pregnancy
by Vicki Iovine (Atria, 2007)

Though it's not enough of a resource guide to help you manage the majority of pregnancy scenarios, this fun and funny read gives great "girlfriend" advice and firsthand stories about life as a pregnant woman. It was by far the most enjoyable book to read during my pregnancy, especially since it didn't inject the fear-factor that's present in so much of today's maternity literature. Drawbacks? Its essay organization requires you do a lot of reading to get at the good tips, and the author is anti-exercise during pregnancy.

Go to Guides for Guys: ABCs for Expectant Dads
by Todd Barrett Lieman (Dalmatian Press, 2007)

Of all the expecting fathers I know, only one actually read any pregnancy book—even though all of them were given a guide that offered perspective on their half of the pregnancy. If it makes you feel better, go ahead and give the soon-to-be-daddies in your life this literature. I promise you that if there is any book that can compel your partner to sit down for a cover-to-cover read, it's this hysterical, extremely male-minded A–Z guide.

Baby Center
www.babycenter.com

This big mama site has all of the pre-pregnancy stuff (think ovulation calculator), pregnancy details (you can track baby's development and learn about the legalities of maternity and paternity leave), and parenting particulars (including weekly e-mails with advice by week, month, and year). You'll find bulletin boards of moms bantering on almost every topic and practically everything else your pregnant mind can conceive of.

iVillage

www.ivillage.com

This women's site is loaded with good pregnancy and parenting info, too, though it takes a bit of a hipper tone and is not as focused as BabyCenter.com (for obvious reasons—not everyone coming here is all about Baby). Still, you'll find lots of tips and ideas for maneuvering through your three trimesters. Another very good resource is its community of birth groups, which you join according to the month of your due date. The benefit is you are all going through the same things at the same time, and it's incredibly reassuring to find out your symptoms, cravings, whatever, are completely normal. There is also a wide variety of experience levels in each group, from first-time moms to old pros, so you can ask any question and someone is bound to either know the answer or how to find it.

Ask Dr. Sears

www.askdrsears.com

This very thorough site is packed with information from the most prolific doctor/wife team in the business. Dr. Bill and Martha Sears are known for their 30+ books on pregnancy and now have a practice with two of their eight children. Their stance is very conventional, so you won't find information about alternative medicine here, but that doesn't diminish the value of its insights, which span from how to finesse pregnancy and beyond.

Mothering

www.mothering.com

This website outpost of the magazine dedicated to natural family living definitely leans toward a groovy parental perspective as is evidenced by articles such as "The Amazing Placenta" and "Sensuous Food for the Mother to Be." But there's also a lot of concrete information for women interested in natural pregnancy, childbirth, and parenting. Though finding the content requires some sniffing around the site, there's some really good stuff here, including details on what's happening with your body and baby each month, miscarriage guidance, Q&As with doctors such as Michel Odent (one of names you hear a lot when talking about natural pregnancies and childbirth), and discussion boards full of interesting banter.

March of Dimes

www.marchofdimes.com

There's a wealth of serious information here, including basic tips, the latest details on premature births, common complications, STDs, what kinds of harmful things to avoid, miscarriage, and even breastfeeding. You'll also find fun "toolkits" like monthly illustrations and written details of how your baby is growing.

BIRTHING

The Birth That's Right for You

1st edition, by Amen Ness, MD; Lisa Gould Rubin, CD, CCR; and Jackie Frederick-Berner (McGraw-Hill, 2005)

What I like about this book is it doesn't tell you that there is one right way to give birth. It neutrally explains all of the possible scenarios, options, and forks in the path, and the authors—an OB-GYN and a doula—spell out everything in layman terms. Even if you know your preferred delivery room direction, a quick read will make you more informed about what actually happens during the last step before motherhood.

About

www.about.com

If you don't want to or can't attend childbirth classes, you can do them online through this site. Check it out even if you are planning to attend a program, as the information is solid and you really can't be too prepared.

The Thinking Woman's Guide to a Better Birth

by Henci Goer (Berkeley Publishing Group, 1999)

A Mommy Menagerie member who is also a delivery nurse told me about this book after I had my baby. It was definitely an unsettling read because it made me realize how little I knew about my birthing choices when I had my daughter—and that had I known more I may have made different decisions. Written by a birth activist (also a doula), it challenges many of today's common medically directed birthing practices, backs up those challenges with medical studies, and helps the reader to understand her options and avoid unnecessary restrictions (like eating while in labor), drugs (epidurals), and procedures (think C-sections and episiotomies). Justified or not, it's really biased toward natural childbirth and against common medical opinion and practice, so if you're planning to go the doctor and hospital route and are thinking of reading this book, know that it can scare you and make you second-guess your choices.

Birth Plan

www.birthplan.com

This site has an interactive tool that allows you to design your birth plan and have it e-mailed to you. Keep in mind that it definitely leans toward minimal medical intervention, so you won't find an option that emphatically demands, "Gimme the drugs the second I walk in the hospital door!" But even if your intention is to take the path of least resistance, filling out the questionnaire will make you aware of some important options and questions, like who will cut the cord, whether you want to watch the birth if you have a C-section, and that you can request to hold your baby before he or she is whisked off to be cleaned and weighed.

Birthing Methods

Lamaze
www.Lamaze.org

Bradley
www.Bradleybirth.com

Hypnobirthing
www.Hypnobirthing.com

Birthing from Within
www.birthingfromwithin.com

Water Birthing
www.Waterbirth.org

ALTERNATIVE PREGNANCY

The Complete Organic Pregnancy

by Deirdre Dolan and Alexandra Zissu (Collins, 2006)

If you're all about the absolute healthiest environment for your fetus and baby, check out this book. It outlines practically every possible toxin in our everyday world, including those in food, water, makeup, furnishings, clothing, cleaning products, pacifiers, and bottles, and offers healthier alternatives. Yes, it's zealous and will make you feel as though your entire home is one big toxic dump. But if you take a moderate attitude and do what you can, this book will empower you to make practical healthy choices for you and your baby.

MULTIPLES

When You're Expecting Twins, Triplets, or Quads

Revised Edition: Proven Guidelines for a Healthy Multiple Pregnancy, by Barbara Luke and Tamara Eberlein (Collins, 2004)

I admit I don't know the first thing about being pregnant with multiples, but I do have several friends with twins. I asked them which book they turned to and they pointed to this one, as did many mommies within their twins club.

National Organization of Mothers of Twins Clubs

www.nomotc.org

A network of more than 450 local clubs representing over 25,000 individual parents of multiples (including triplets, quadruplets, and beyond), this organization doesn't have tons of information on its site, but it is practiced at connecting expecting parents with local clubs. It also has a section with lots of links, and great members-only bulletin boards.

Mothers of Supertwins

www.mostonline.org

This is an international support organization for parents of triplets and up (a.k.a. "higher order multiples"). You have to pay $25 to join the organization and access its online forums and receive its magazine, but you can browse a FAQ page that gives brief answers to questions ranging from "What are the odds of having a multiple birth?" to "How much weight will I gain while pregnant with higher-order multiples?"

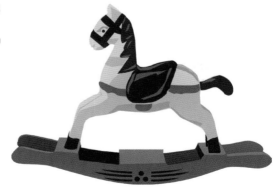

Maternity and Paternity Leave

Department of Labor

www.dol.gov

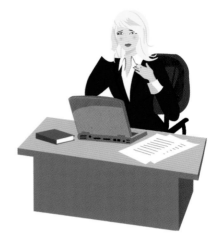

Don't know your rights as a pregnant mother or expecting father in the workplace? Go to this governmental site, click on "Search / A to Z Index" in the upper right hand corner, and type "maternity leave" or paternity leave" into the search box, and you'll get all the details on The Family and Medical Leave Act of 1993, which outlines your eligibility, leave entitlement, and more.

Exercise

BabyFit

www.babyfit.com

Truth is, I couldn't find one genuine rock star pregnancy exercise book or website. But this one did a decent job of covering maternity fitness, is free, and allows you to set up your own fitness profile. The Resource Center, which is accessed by a tiny link at the bottom of the home page, actually has tons of information, including exercise demos and tips on how to stay safe during workouts and ease symptoms and discomforts and post-pregnancy fitness. Added bonus: The message boards here are very current.

High-Risk Pregnancy

Sidelines

www.sidelines.org

The site for the National High Risk Pregnancy Support Network posts good articles on a variety of subjects, offers tons of links to resources for all the different kinds of high risks, and even has a downloadable bedrest checklist.

Pregnancy Loss

Share

www.nationalshareoffice.com

There are tons of sites offering support for pregnancy losses, but many of them have religious, spiritual, or touchy-feely angles to them. I chose to include this one because it has an enormous amount of information and support, regularly occurring online chats, and an even tone that will appeal to the broadest range of grieving mothers. Check it out and also search the web for sites that you best identify with.

SHOPPING

Baby Bargains

7th Edition: Secrets to Saving 20% to 50% on Baby Furniture, Gear, Clothes, Toys, Maternity Wear and Much More! (Windsor Peak Press, 2007)

You will need help navigating all of the baby gear options and this book is the one to give it to you. It reviews loads of popular brands, offers arguments on stuff to buy and stuff to skip, and provides secrets on how to shave hundreds of dollars off the bottom line. I didn't have this when I was pregnant, but if I did it might have stopped me from constantly quizzing all of my mommy friends.

POSTPARTUM

Postpartum

www.postpartum.net

This nice, sleek, and soothing site run by an international organization was founded to "eliminate denial and ignorance of emotional health related to childbirth." If your new life has you feeling blue, drop by here and check out the resources section for great articles, their bookstore for helpful literature on the subject, and their Support Groups and Area Coordinators tab for help near you.

PARENTHOOD

What to Expect the First Year

2nd edition, by Heidi Murkoff, Sandee Hathaway, and Arlene Eisenberg (Workman Publishing, 2004)

Though a good all-around reference book for baby milestones and basic information on everything from breastfeeding to common illnesses to burping and sleeping, the month-by-month organization deems what your baby should be able to do at a certain time and can freak out parents whose child is not going by the book so to speak. Still, it's a hefty and decent reference to have around the house so long as you know that life doesn't always go according to an author's plan.

Healthy Sleep Habits, Happy Child

by Marc Weissbluth (Ballantine Books, 2005)

As I mentioned earlier in this book you don't want to start thinking about how to help your restless bundle of joy get some beauty sleep when you're bleary-eyed and desperate for answers. This book doesn't unlock all of the secrets to good sleeping routines. In fact, on more than one occasion I yearned for more guidance (like when at 15 months my daughter dropped her afternoon nap instead of her morning one). But it does give enough guidelines and information to help you get your little one into a groove, which is essential for a joyful baby and sane parents. Just keep in mind that advice books are just that: advice. You know your baby best and should always go with your gut.

Breastfeeding

The Nursing Mother's Companion

5th edition, by Kathleen Huggins (Harvard Common Press, 2005)

If you're planning to breastfeed, don't make the mistake of thinking that just because your jugs are full you'll have an easy time pouring the milk. This book, which is overflowing with good advice, troubleshooting tips, and even details on the best breast pump, will prepare you for the practicalities and problems before they arise.

Dr. Jack Newman

www.drjacknewman.com

If you begin breastfeeding, encounter problems, and are committed to keeping it up, you will find yourself frantically searching for anyone and everyone who can offer you advice. Check this online breastfeeding resource by a pediatrician and board-certified lactation consultant. It is robust and has video demos of proper and improper latches and other mammary maneuvers, plus access to local support.

Got Mom

www.gotmom.org

Another excellent breastfeeding source, this site is by the American College of Nurse-Midwives in association with Avent Naturally, the baby bottle, pacifier, and pump company. Like all breastfeeding sites, it's definitely pro going with the flow. Stop by for breastfeeding tips, a list of good books to read, the latest news and research, and resources for getting help.

Kelly Mom

www.kellymom.com

Yet another source for your nursing needs, this one also includes information on postpartum depression, parenting, and books. It also has a forum, handouts, and fun polls.

International Lactation Consultant Association

www.ilca.com

That's right. Lactation consulting is in such high demand there's an actual association of nationwide professionals. Good thing, too, because if you ever need one you'll be delighted to have local resources at your fingertips. Just pop your zip code into their nifty search engine and you'll get a list of available help near you.

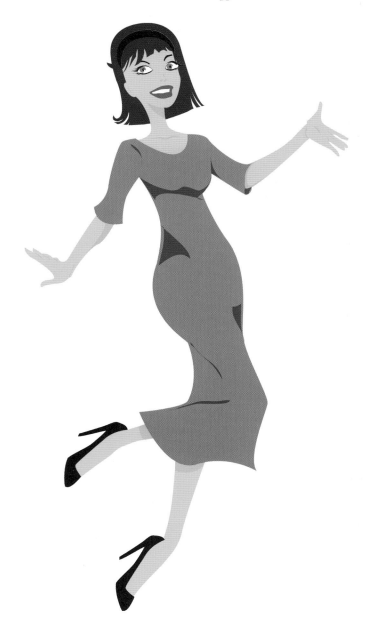

Author's Ackowledgments

As a mother I can't help but laugh when authors say that writing a book is like having a baby. Clearly, they haven't lugged around a human basketball during the hottest summer months or doubled over with the pains of labor. As you will soon attest, absolutely nothing compares to giving birth or the miraculous process that leads up to it.

Penning this primer was a different sort of labor of love inspired by my own pregnancy. Only there were way more than two people involved in its conception and final delivery, and all of them deserve a celebratory cigar, enthusiastic pat on the back, and enormous thank you.

First and foremost I must give props to my husband Colie Wertz. I literally couldn't have done it without him. Also huge thanks to my brilliant agent, friend, and literary coach Carole Bidnick, who championed this book as if it were her own baby and continues to be one of my most knowledgeable and trusted professional confidants.

I've been in the business long enough to know that publisher support is about as guaranteed as your baby being born on its due date, so it's impossible to express the extent of gratitude and appreciation I have for the entire DK team, starting with my editor and pal Anja Schmidt. She was so committed to this book she actually got pregnant before I turned it in just so she could make sure it accurately addressed all the critical topics. (Okay, maybe that wasn't the first reason she got pregnant, but our publishing partnership was kismet and her friendship and input has been invaluable.) Notable nods also go to assistant editor Nichole Morford, who took the editorial torch and ran with it like an Olympian sprinter when Anja went on maternity leave, and to talented managing art editor Michelle Baxter, who graciously fielded my endless comments and still had time to create a gloriously colorful and approachable platform for my words. Also eternal thanks to editorial head Sharon Lucas and marketing guru Judi Powers for getting behind me and this book, and publicity manager Rachael Kempster for helping to get the word out.

Then there's the Mommy Menagerie, the group of 111 women from all over the country and abroad who generously shared their most private pregnancy experiences. This book would not be nearly as insightful, honest, and helpful without them and I am beyond honored by their contribution. You'll find a list of the fabulous women that gave me permission to give them a shout out by name on the following two pages.

I also want to throw my hands in the air and wave 'em like I just don't care for Dr. Susan L. Sterlacci, the highly respected and knowledgeable New York OB-GYN who diligently poured over these pages to make sure my research and advice didn't miss a medical beat. Ditto my dear friend Lyla Max who helped organize and sort the abundant data imparted by the Mommy Menagerie and was my go-to girl every time I had a question about how to handle my newborn. I'm also sending a heaping helping of plate-licking props to the culinary greats who contributed tasty cravings recipes. José Ramón Andrés, Bertrand Bouquin, Katie Brown, Josiah Citrin, Cat Cora, Ruta Kahate, Trish Karter, Cindi Kruth, and Dana Slatkin, this means you!

This book would be nothing but blank pages if it weren't for my friend Geny Ceh, who helped me care for my daughter and myself while I was on deadline, taught me a tremendous amount about motherhood, and whipped up insanely good chicken taquitos when I needed them most. Likewise Yesenia Arvizu who shared diaper, playground, and baby-coddling duty.

Finally, a major hug and big smooch to my mother, Faith Winthrop, who I now appreciate in ways I could never have before I was a mom. Thanks for toting me around in your innards for nine months and raising me to believe that I can do anything. My success in life has everything to do with you.

ACKNOWLEDGMENTS

THE MOMMY MENAGERIE

Some of these women I know, but most of the 111 women referred to in this book as the Mommy Menagerie are complete strangers that found me through online bulletin board postings or forwarded e-mails from friends of friends. The ages during which they were pregnant range from 18 to 45 and their hometowns span across the states, Canada, and Europe.

Besides being mothers, the one thing all of these wondrous femmes have in common is that they were kind enough to fill out my laborious 68-question survey to help bring a spectacular variety of genuine, experiential truths to this book.

Behold the magnificent Mommy Menagerie, whose humor, humanity, tips, and anecdotes are sprinkled throughout *The Real Deal Guide to Pregnancy*.

- Amanda Aaronson
- Jennifer Aaronson
- Jessica Abbott
- Nichole Accetolla
- Carlye Adler-Fieldman
- Heather Ames
- Holly A. Ames
- Steffani Aranas
- Kristy Ashbaucher
- Katie Baird
- Lisa Barnes
- Lori Barrett
- Leslie Bauer
- Isabelle Bax Finney
- Tida Beattie
- Faith Begay-Holtrop
- Michelle Berney
- Shannah Biggs
- Lisa Blankespoor
- Sharon Cain
- Michaela Calanchini-Carter
- Connie Castellino

- Karen Causey Williams
- Jessica Colvin
- Naomi Crawford
- Lori Dalvi
- Shamini Dhana
- Edie Dillman
- Brooke Dorman
- Wendy Downing
- Victoria Emery
- Amalia Egri Freedman
- Heidi Ernst Jones
- Suzanne Esser
- Elizabeth Flemming
- Catharine Freyer
- Mary "from Vermont"
- Alexandra Galanter
- Kristi Galarneau
- Amy Goodwin
- RuthAnn Goradia
- Misty Griffis
- Tracy Guth Spangler
- Maggie Harmon

- Margo Hays
- Lynda Hess
- Penelope Hoblyn
- Jennifer Hix
- Anita Jackson
- Rebecca Jackson
- Cynthia James
- Denise Keller
- Lisa Kendrick
- Julie Kessler
- Leslie Kline
- Maria Koronatova Ralph
- Petrona Kral
- Dawn Larkin
- Melissa Lee
- Candice Lenkowsky
- Karen Lewis
- Kristen Lewis
- Annie Longsworth
- Karen Manuel
- Kelly Martin
- Tammy McConaughy

- Tracy McGillis
- Marion McKee
- Kate McMahon
- Cindy McSherry-Martinez
- Mary Meehan
- Brigette Miller
- Ashlie Moore
- Bethany Mutone
- Gina Pell
- Natasha Persad
- Carrie Piccard
- Kimberly Postlewaite
- Courtney Price

- Lisa Reagan Parker
- Alexandra Reuter
- Renee Robinett
- Jenny Rohde
- Joanna Russo
- Alexandra Sanidad Zangrillo
- Deedee Schiano
- Samantha Schoech
- Diane Schoonover
- Veronica Skelton
- Ingrid Sperow
- Samantha Steinwinder
- Debra Talwalkar

- Suzanne Tavolacci
- Jennifer Toland
- Heather Toll
- Lisa Vance
- Angie Wagner
- Elizabeth A. Walls
- Noel Weimer
- Kristin White-Slye
- Meg Wilson
- Kate Winslow
- Julie Wright
- Jen Zagofsky
- Jennifer Zimmerman

DK's Acknowledgments

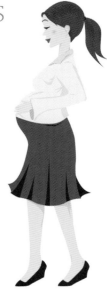

DK would like to thank:

Nicole Turney for her proofreading skills.

Nanette Cardon for her speedy indexing.

Top Notch for color proofing.

Diana Catherines for rushing to the delivery room at the

last minute and producing endless illustrations and revisions.

And Leofwin Muskin for arriving at the perfect time.